RELEASED

NUTRITION
COUNSELING
SKILLS

Assessment, Treatment, and Evaluation

Linda G. Snetselaar, R.D., Ph.D.

Lipid Research Clinic
University of Iowa

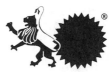

AN ASPEN PUBLICATION®
Aspen Systems Corporation
Rockville, Maryland
London
1983

Library of Congress Cataloging in Publication Data

Snetselaar, Linda G.
Nutrition counseling skills.

Includes bibliographical references and index.
1. Obesity—Psychological aspects.
2. Health counseling. I. Title
[DNLM: 1. Nutrition. 2. Counseling. QU 145 S67in]
RC628.S646   1983   616.3'98'0019   83-9932
ISBN: 0-89443-880-8

Publisher: John Marozsan
Editorial Director: Darlene Como
Executive Managing Editor: Margot Raphael
Editorial Services: Scott Ballotin
Printing and Manufacturing: Debbie Collins

Library of Congress Catalog Card Number 83-9932
ISBN: 0-89443-880-8

Printed in the United States of America

3   4   5

To my husband
Gary

Table of Contents

fast

Foreword

Nutrition has tremendous potential for the prevention and treatment of disease throughout the life cycle. As science advances, more becomes known about food, its components, and its value for health promotion. Research to identify more efficient and effective means to disseminate information about nutrition to the health professions and the public is under way.

An increased awareness of the value of nutrition in prevention and treatment of such major diseases as obesity, hyperlipidemia, hypertension, and diabetes is coupled with the demand that nutrition education efforts be increased and the results improved. Nutrition educators and counselors are increasing their capabilities as nutrition counselors by enrolling in university-based courses and continuing education activities such as workshops sponsored by the American Dietetic Association; the American Heart Association; and the National Heart, Lung, and Blood Institute, National Institutes of Health. In addition, publications to assist with the educational programs are increasing. All of these efforts should assist nutrition counselors to become more effective and to increase the use of nutritional measures for both the prevention and treatment of disease.

Marilyn Farrand, R.D.
Public Health Nutritionist

Preface

This book is designed to help nutrition counselors perform their jobs more effectively. The term nutrition counselor is used to describe all health professionals involved in counseling clients or patients in dietary instructions and adherence, either generally (Chapters 1 through 3) or in cases where medical factors necessitate changes in eating habits (Chapters 4 through 10). Thus, nutrition counselors may be registered dietitians or they may be other health professionals—medical doctors, nurses, psychologists, or behavior therapists—who work with registered dietitians.

Both interviewing and counseling skills, including examples of how nutrition counselors might apply those capabilities, are discussed. Reader goals include acquiring or enhancing the ability:

1. to demonstrate effective use of interviewing skills
2. to select and apply appropriate strategies when presented with nutrition problems
3. to evaluate progress, achievements, and failures in both clients and self
4. to adapt counseling strategies based on self-evaluations and client evaluations.

Nutrition Counseling Skills was written to supplement a major course in nutrition principles. Its intent is to (1) apply interviewing and counseling skills and strategies to the discipline of nutrition and (2) provide for their practice in situations where specific diet modifications are mandated. Ideally this work should be supplemented by a course in counseling psychology.

This does not replace discussions on basic nutrition principles and none of the information will be useful without a thorough understanding of that subject as taught in a college curriculum. This work is designed as a supplement to current practices in nutrition counseling.

Each chapter begins with an outline of topics presented and concludes with a list of reference material for further study. Part I covers basic theories on interviewing and counseling skills. Part II demonstrates how those skills may be practiced in specific nutrition situations where eating behaviors may pose problems.

The term "eating pattern" is used frequently instead of "diet" to get away from a term that implies adherence one day and nonadherence the next day. "Diet" tends to denote following an eating regimen, then going back to old habits.

All exhibits, figures, and tables not otherwise credited are by the author.

Linda G. Snetselaar
August 1983

Acknowledgments

The author acknowledges the expertise of those without whose help this book would not have been possible:

Barry Bratton, Ph.D.
Jacqueline Dunbar, Ph.D.
Harold Engen, Ed.D.
Kathryn Mahoney, Ph.D.
Helmut Schrott, M.D.
Karen Smith, R.D., M.S.
Rhonda Dale Terry, Ph.D.
Laura Vailas, R.D., M.S.

Appendix H, the Lipid Research Clinic Food Substitution Guide project at the University of Iowa in 1977, was funded in part by the Lipid Research Clinic, Coronary Primary Prevention Trial, and the National Heart, Lung, and Blood Institute, for which the author expresses deep appreciation.

Special thanks go to Beverly Kuddes and Sandra Breland for their labors during their free time in typing this manuscript.

Finally, this book would not have been possible without the interest and enthusiasm of Marilyn Farrand. Her innovative approaches to dietetic practices have supported the idea of applying counseling skills to the dissemination of nutrition information.

Part I

Basic Theories in Interviewing and Counseling Skills

This part covers basic ideas on the theoretical aspects of interviewing and counseling skills in relation to nutrition and eating behaviors. Terms used in the field are discussed. (They also are defined in the glossary.)

Each chapter begins with a list of objectives for readers. Each ends with a list of references for more in-depth reading, particularly on some topics that may be covered only peripherally in the text.

Overview of Nutrition Counseling

Objectives for Chapter 1

1. Discuss the influence of counseling theory on the client.
2. Describe three theories that influence the nutrition counselor.
3. Discuss two ways in which counseling is important to the work of the nutrition counselor.
4. Identify the components of counseling skills.
5. Draw the counseling spectrum.

1

DEFINITION OF NUTRITION COUNSELING

Nutrition has been described as both a science and an art. The nutrition counselor's goals are to convert theory into practice and science into art. This ability requires a great deal of knowledge and skill.[1]

Nutrition is a profession requiring knowledge of diverse subjects and counselors in the field must be well versed in many areas, including biochemistry, physiology, botany, and agriculture. To use this knowledge to change food behaviors, they also must have an understanding of the art of helping others, the art of counseling.

What is nutrition counseling? Mason et al. define it as "helping people with present or potential nutrition problems, whether they exist because of lack of knowledge, or motivation, or both."[2]

HISTORY OF NUTRITION COUNSELING

Over the years nutrition advice has been a part of nearly every culture. Early Greek physicians recognized the role of food in the treatment of disease.[3] In America in the early 1800s Thomas Jefferson described his eating habits in a letter to his doctor in what may be one of the first diet records.[4] (Exhibit 1–1) After World War II, advances in chemical knowledge allowed nutrition researchers to define metabolic requirements.[5] This marked the beginning of looking at patterns of nutrients needed by all persons in relation to their age, sex, and activity. These patterns are vital to what is termed the assessment phase of counseling.

5

Exhibit 1–1 A Colonial Era Diet Report

"... I have lived temperately, eating little animal food, ... except as a condiment for vegetables, which constitute my principle diet. I double, however, the doctor's glass and a half of wine."

From Thomas Jefferson
to his Doctor

Source: The Thomas Jefferson Memorial Foundation, Monticello, Charlottesville, Va.

Selling and Ferraro, in discussing the psychology of diet and nutrition in 1945, recommended what, at that time, must have been a rather unconventional view:

1. knowing the client's personality
2. knowing the client's psychological surroundings
3. eliminating emotional tension
4. assisting the client in knowing his own limitations
5. arranging the diet so that it has the effect of encouraging the client
6. allowing for occasional cheating [on the diet].[6]

Practitioners can recognize the value of these suggestions, but are they followed routinely today?

Nutrition advice has changed over the years as described in terms of the counselors' roles during a session. In the past, the role fell more on the authoritarian side of a continuum; today, all roles are necessary for optimum performance (Figure 1–1).

Pioneers in the Field

One of the first pioneers in nutrition counseling, Margaret Ohlson, in 1973 stressed the importance of creating an interviewing atmosphere in which the client can respond freely. This can occur only when the counselor's listening skills are attuned to hearing what the client is saying. Ohlson warns against what is a common problem in dietetic counseling sessions: speaking at the expense of missing important factors during the interview.[7]

Selling and Ferraro say there no longer is any justification for prescribing a diet without also recognizing the psychological factors in a case. They recommend that a diagnostic study be made to determine the right psychodietetic approach.[8]

Figure 1–1 Roles of the Nutrition Counselor Today

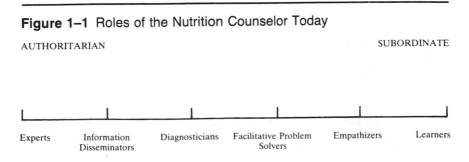

AUTHORITARIAN   SUBORDINATE

| Experts | Information Disseminators | Diagnosticians | Facilitative Problem Solvers | Empathizers | Learners |

Theories Influence Clients

As in every discipline, several theories from the past have formed the basis for developing the counseling skills of nutrition practitioners and other health professionals responsible for patient education and have led them to view counseling as a means of changing eating habits. Both clients and counselors use theories and beliefs in determining what will take place during an interview.

Clients approach nutrition counseling sessions with mind-sets about themselves and the world around them. They present "a history of being healed or hurt by others, of being accepted or rejected, of dominating others or treating them as equals, of seeing people as ends or means."[9] They also come with a positive or negative self-image and with a record of success or failure in diet modification. From this stems their personal theories of what counseling is and should be.

Most practitioners have faced a client who slouches down in the chair, slams a diet instruction sheet on the desk, and demands: "Well, what are you going to do to get me to follow this diet?" This client sees the counselor as an expert, the person with all of the answers—and an adversary. A second client may walk into the office, sit down, and from that time on speak only when spoken to. Still a third client will arrive commenting, "Well, how can we work out this problem I've been having with my diet?"

All three clients see the world through different eyes. The first does not want any responsibility, the second may be afraid of authority figures, and the last sees the counselor as an advocate, as someone who can help increase self-directed solutions to problems with diet.

Lorr lists five descriptors of client perception of counselors:

1. accepting
2. understanding
3. independence-encouraging
4. authoritarian
5. critical-hostile.[10]

Clients may be programmed before the interview to see the nutrition counselor as rejecting, dominating, and hostile. Consequently, they will resort to behavior they have used in the past in dealing with that sort of unapproachable person. Other clients, on the basis of past experience, may see counselors as friendly, supportive, respectful, and positive. Both of these situations could create self-fulfilling prophecies. Counselors could become trapped into behaving in accordance with the clients' theory of the world.

Clients also come to a nutrition counseling session with feelings about self. They want to succeed in changing, yet at the same time seek to sabotage any efforts toward change so their routines will stay the same.[11] Clients say, "New eating habits may be healthy but what changes will they make in my family life?" A familiar overweight image can give obese persons a sense of identity and security that they could lose when the pounds come off. Some clients comment, "People expect less of me this way. Why should I change that secure feeling I have to a feeling of having to shape up to what people want me to be?"

Clients come to counseling with

1. attitudes and beliefs about people
2. ideas and feelings about counselors and counseling
3. self images, and
4. basic incongruities in desired outcomes:
   - wanting to continue along a familiar course, and
   - on the other hand, wanting to make changes to improve health and well-being.[12]

Counseling is a skill used to correct or validate clients' preconceived beliefs. It is a skill that enables counselors to behave as decent, empathic persons in spite of the "provocation to be less or the seduction to be more" than they are.[13]

Theories Influence Counselors

There are many different theories that can influence the way in which a nutrition counselor conducts a session and they can be categorized in many different ways. A shortened version of four of the theories is:

1. client-centered therapy
2. rational emotive therapy (RET)
3. behavioral therapy
4. Gestalt therapy

Their characteristics as they might apply directly to the nutrition counseling session are analyzed next. It should be noted that ideas in many of these theories overlap.

Client-Centered Therapy

Carl Rogers is the founder of the first theory, client-centered therapy.[14] It is based on three major concepts.

1. All individuals are a composite of their physical being, their thoughts, and their behaviors.
2. Individuals function as an organized system, so alterations in one part may produce changes in another part.
3. Individuals react to everything they perceive; this is their reality.

When counselors try to change dietary behaviors, they also must be concerned with clients' thoughts. Behavioral alterations may produce changes in the clients' physical being as well as the cognitive (thoughtful) being. It also is necessary to be very thorough in assessing client perceptions because what is perceived as reality influences ability to follow the diet.

The goals of client-centered therapy include:

1. promoting a more confident and self-directed person
2. promoting a more realistic self-perception, and
3. promoting a positive attitude about self.[15]

Nutrition counselors should provide the tools to help clients solve their own problems through assessing their current dietary behavior and establishing realistic goals for change. Practitioners also can assess clients' thoughts about their body image and food behaviors. Changing thoughts from negative to positive can go a long way in helping the obese.

Rational Emotive Therapy

The second theory, rational emotive therapy (RET), was developed by Albert Ellis. He determined that irrationality was the most frequent source of individuals' problems and self-talk (the monologues individuals carry on with themselves) the major cause of emotion-related difficulties.[16] This theory's major purposes are to demonstrate to clients that self-talk is the source of their problems and that they should reevaluate it in order to eliminate it and illogical ideas.[17] The clients' major goal is to look to self for positive reinforcement for behaviors.

In dietary counseling, an overweight client says:

"I knew I shouldn't eat that piece of pie, but I did. After eating it, I decided, well, what's the use, you've been such a bad person for eating it. You're just making yourself fat and ugly. It's no use. So I ate the entire pie."

The counselor in this case can help change self-talk to more positive thoughts: "I ate one piece. Even if it was high in calories, I don't need to feel guilty. I won't eat another piece and that's great. I'm really doing well. I feel better about myself."

Behavioral Therapy

Behavioral counseling can be traced back to several theorists: Pavlov, Skinner, Wolpe, Krumboltz, and Thoreson. This theory states that people are born into this world in a neutral state. Environment, consisting of significant others and experience, shapes their behavior.

Three modes of learning are basic to behavioral counseling:[18]

1. *Operant Conditioning:* If spontaneous behavior satisfies a need, this conduct will occur with greater frequency. For example, a person who switches to a high-fiber diet finds that constipation problems are reduced. As a result, this client probably will increase the fiber in all meals.
2. *Imitation:* This does not involve teaching a new behavior; instead, the emphasis is on mimicking. The overweight client selects a low-calorie snack after a spouse or friend has just ordered one in a restaurant.
3. *Modeling:* This extends the concept of imitation, which tends to be haphazard, by providing a planned demonstration. Modeling implies direct teaching of a certain behavior.[19] An overweight client watches a videotape of someone who has just lost a large amount of weight. The model's description or demonstration of successful weight loss behaviors should provide impetus for the client to begin a weight-loss program.

The goals of behavioral counseling obviously will vary with each client.

Gestalt Therapy

This type of counseling emphasizes confronting problems. Steps toward solving problems involve experience in the present rather than the past or the future.

The major goal in Gestalt therapy is to bring into the clients' awareness all experience that they have disowned, along with the recognition that individuals are self-regulating. Being aware of hidden factors related to a problem is the key to finding an eventual solution.[20]

Helping obese clients recognize how many "disowned" factors can contribute to their overweight problems and showing how to be responsible for regulating behavior is a practical application of the Gestalt approach to counseling.

In practice, most counselors use a combination of these theories, "a kind of reasoned eclecticism."[21] Given the reality of dealing with an individual client, the counselor must rise above the principles of abstract theory and must apply strategies most appropriate for that person.

IMPORTANCE OF NUTRITION COUNSELING

Why is counseling important? For years the profession has survived without worrying about how abstract theories affect clients and counselors, so why worry about it now?

Dietary Adherence

One very important reason why counseling skills are an important part of a nutrition interview is dietary adherence, i.e., how well clients follow practitioners' recommendations. Research has shown that there are many deterrents to dietary adherence:

1. the restrictiveness of the dietary pattern
2. the required changes in life style and behavior
3. the symptom relief may not be noticeable or may be temporary
4. diets may interfere with family or personal habits, and
5. other barriers
   - Cost
   - Access to proper foods, and
   - Effort necessary for food preparation.[22]

In this same study, Glanz shows that there appear to be many positive counseling techniques that increase dietary adherence:

1. employing more strategies which influence client behavior,
2. involving clients more during the session.[23]

Hosking lists conditions that increase dietary adherence in hypertensive clients on salt-restricted eating patterns:

1. diet programs that are individualized, fully explained, and adapted to the client's preferences and life style,
2. regular revisits and seeing the same nutrition counselor on each visit,
3. involvement of the family, and

4. reinforcement of the eating pattern from every member of the treatment team.[24]

Several research studies have shown that better adherence results when the counselor is warm and empathetic and shows interest ("Call me if there is a problem") and demonstrates genuine concern ("I will call in a week").[25,26,27,28,29]

A second important reason for considering counseling skills an important part of nutrition practice is that they can help eliminate the hit-or-miss philosophy that allows no assurance for success. This philosophy also tends to be inefficient because the nutrition counselor must backtrack when strategies fail. To provide structure and organization many counseling models such as the following have been suggested.[30,31,32]

Systems Approach to Nutrition Counseling

Models provide a sequenced path for counselors to follow. They list essential components in each step of the process. Figure 1–2 shows one model by which nutrition counselors can avoid missing a vital part of the process.

In this model the counselor wears many hats. The first role is that of a diagnostician preparing for the interview by reviewing all available data in the medical record.

The session begins with an explanation of the counseling relationship with enough description so that the client knows precisely what will take place. In this role the practitioner is a teacher informing the client of what the relationship is.

During the assessment phase, once again in the role of diagnostician, the counselor evaluates the client's nutrition status and relates food intake data to behavioral indicators. The practitioner also must establish a safe, trusting, and caring environment, acting as empathizer.

Mason specifies the categories of information necessary for assessment of clients' nutritional status:

1. agricultural data
2. socioeconomic data
3. food consumption patterns
4. dietary surveys
5. special studies on foods
6. vital and health statistics
7. anthropometric studies
8. clinical nutrition survey

Figure 1–2 Model for Nutrition Counseling

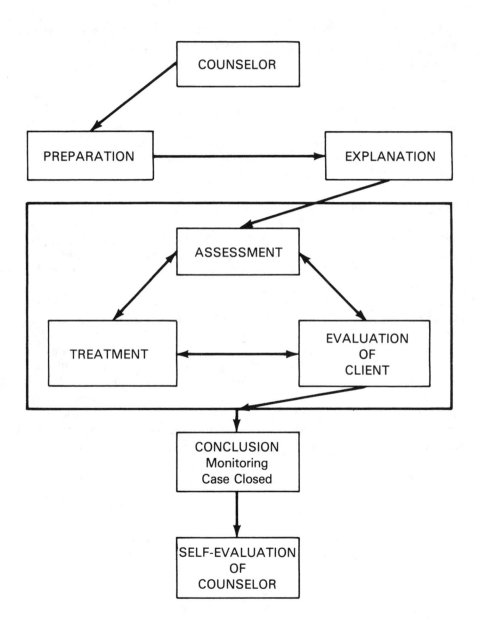

9. biochemical studies
10. additional medical information.[33]

Information is also necessary to assess behavior. Mason designates several categories in determining baseline behaviors:

1. general health practices
2. health, attitudes, beliefs and information
3. physical activities
4. educational achievements and language skills
5. economic considerations
6. environmental considerations
7. social considerations.[34]

In the treatment phase, the roles are those of expert and mutual problem solver. These can be very difficult roles to combine and can be achieved only through diligent study and practice. Most novices at counseling tend to fall into one of these categories—expert or empathizer. Neither role is bad when the two are used in combination but when performed singly, each can be detrimental to effective counseling.

Many practitioners are familiar with the all-knowing counselor who approaches clients with an air of authority. The clients are overwhelmed by these experts' self-confidence and are taken in by the appearance of wisdom. However, when clients return home, they find it very difficult to follow the diet. They tend to forget much of what was said during the counseling session and are incapable of self-direction in adhering to the new regimen. The clients' solution in such a case is to continue with old eating habits.

On the other hand, the mutual problem solvers can become so involved with client problems that sight is lost of the other role as information disseminators. Counselors can run into conflicts when it is apparent that the clients are in error but feel that revealing the mistake may damage the individuals' pride and ability to follow the diet.

"Eating fried shrimp out a few times won't matter," the counselor says. To the client on a low-cholesterol diet this may be a signal to go ahead and continue poor eating habits. Back at home, the client may comment to a family member, "The nutritionist said eating shrimp in a restaurant just a few times wouldn't hurt. Three nights a week doesn't seem too often."

In evaluating clients, counselors once again become diagnosticians. If no solution to the problem has been reached, counseling reverts to the assessment or treatment phase. In some cases the clinicians may decide to refer a client to another practitioner more experienced with the problem. In such a case the new counselor probably would start from the beginning.

In concluding the counseling session, work with the clients should be on a mutual basis with possibly a few notes of wisdom, in which case the counselors become the experts again. Ending the program involves more than just closing the case. Monitoring the clients' performance in the real world is important to continued dietary adherence. This means calling to check on progress and, with the individual's permission, checking with significant others to determine how they feel the clients have progressed.

The last step involves self-evaluation of the counselors' performance. In this case the counselors become the learners, building on past experience to improve present skills.

COUNSELING SKILLS

What skills are involved in counseling? The basic steps just discussed are part of it but counseling is much more complex than Figure 1–2 (supra) indicates. (Chapters 2 and 3 review these skills and ways to use them.)

Interviewing Skills

Basic to all counseling is a knowledge of interviewing skills. Without these, treatment cannot and will not take place.

Counseling Skills

Once clinicians have acquired this foundation, they then can learn various counseling skills to aid clients in achieving dietary goals. These skills involve assessment, treatment (including planning and implementation), and evaluation.

Assessment

Assessment involves more than asking clients, "Do you have a problem?" It is a carefully thought out plan to determine areas in which problems occur.

Assessment in nutrition counseling includes ascertaining both what the clients are eating and why certain food selections are made.[35] How do practitioners adequately elicit responses to both of these inquiries?

The example that follows illustrates a problem that occurs particularly with weight-control individuals.

A client returns for a visit following the diet instruction and reports a problem: "I just haven't lost any weight on the diet you recommended." There are several responses:

1. "Did you follow all of my advice?"
2. "Well, what have you been eating?"
3. "What is your typical day like?"

The first question is stated in a way that immediately places clients on the defensive. They feel compelled to give a glowing picture or a multitude of excuses.

The second question focuses only on eating behaviors, disregarding totally the surrounding circumstances that may have instigated the behavior. Depending on the tone of voice, it also may make the clients feel compelled to reply with what the counselors want to hear.

The third question is stated sensitively and with a show of caring. It does not imply a reprimand. It also leaves the clients room to elaborate on what actually happened and gives the counselors the information necessary to assess the situation.

In work with practicing nutrition counselors, the author has found the problem that most frequently occurs during an interview is their rush to give advice. It is important to stop and take time to assess the situation first and only then provide advice, allowing the clients to assist by describing how they expect to apply those recommendations in a true-to-life situation.

Treatment

In providing strategies to remedy nutrition problems or provide treatment, counselors once again must proceed slowly and involve the clients in planning and setting attainable goals. Counselors frequently decide before the interview how the problem should be solved and try to force clients into preformed molds. They do not give the clients an opportunity to participate. In this phase, mutually decided goals will achieve the most success. Counselors should use this sequence of steps in setting goals:

1. Identify nutrition goals
   - Define desired nutrition behaviors [what to do].
   - Determine conditions or circumstances [where and when to do it].
   - Establish the extent or level [how much or how often to do].

2. Identify nutrition subgoals [a subgoal for a long-term goal of eliminating snacks would be to eliminate the morning snack and determine a workable substitute behavior].
3. Establish client commitment.[36]

The strategy chosen to help implement these goals once again requires patient listeners who are willing to involve the clients in reaching solutions. Strategies are numerous and require knowledge and experience in counseling psychology. In deciding on a strategy, counselors should ask these questions:

1. Why is the client here?
2. Is the problem the client describes all or only part of the problem? [Many nutrition counselors have thrown their hands up in despair saying, "He just isn't motivated to follow this diet." In that case the real problem may hinge on emotional stress that must be treated before nutrition counseling can take place. The client might be referred to a psychologist or other professional for help before beginning the nutrition counseling session.]
3. What are the problematic nutrition behaviors and related concerns?
4. Can I describe the conditions contributing to poor nutrition adherence?
5. Am I aware of the present severity and intensity of the nutrition problem?[37]

Numerous types of strategies are presented in Chapter 3. The following three have had the most applicability in the author's work with clients.

The first is self-monitoring, which involves asking the clients to record food intake over a period of three to seven days. This is used most frequently in the assessment phase but it also can provide clients with a review of problem days or times during the day and can result automatically in changed behavior.

The second, modeling, has been suggested for weight control. One example: showing an overweight client a videotape of someone who has gone through a weight-control program. The once overweight model's description of how to overcome the problem may be just what the client needs to feel courageous and confident enough to continue in a program.

The third, a rather new strategy used successfully by Mahoney and Mahoney (1976), is called cognitive restructuring.[38,39] This strategy helps clients think in more positive terms about body image, weight loss, and food in general. Some overweight clients the author has counseled tend to see weight loss as an all-or-nothing game:

"I ate one piece of that high-calorie cheesecake. I knew I shouldn't have done that. I'm such a failure at everything I do. Losing weight is no use. I might as well eat myself sick."

Helping such clients see that occasional variances from the low-calorie prescription are acceptable can be a great step forward in eliminating binge eating behaviors. Dichotomous (all-or-none) thinking tends to push many enthusiastic weight-control individuals into a trap of frustration. It is worthwhile for future dietary maintenance to discuss this thinking process with the clients and point out its pitfalls.

Evaluation

The last phase, evaluation, provides a reassessment of progress for both clients and counselors. Much of the questioning used during the assessment phase can be reused here, focusing on the desired objective and whether or not it was met. The counselors should monitor clients for a time in the real world, asking permission to check with significant others as to whether they feel the persons are doing well.

Counselor self-evaluation frequently does not take place due to time constraints. It can be very important to review what went on in an interview, then determine what made it a success and what might have improved its efficacy or quality.

COUNSELING SPECTRUM

Nutrition counselors, as noted, assume a variety of roles. During the sessions some role changes will take place automatically, others will require a great deal of practice and effort. The role as nutritionists will fall on a spectrum such as that in Figure 1–3, including some of the positions on both ends. When counseling is totally dominated by client requests and tangential topics, little behavior change will take place. A session totally dominated by counselors who provide only information, without listening

Figure 1–3 The Nutrition Counseling Spectrum

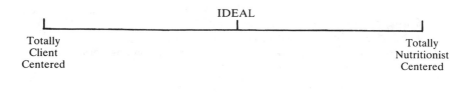

to client concerns, can be equally unproductive. The ideal is a mix of client and counselor interaction.

NOTES

1. Marion Mason, Burness G. Wenberg, and P. Kay Welch, *The Dynamics of Clinical Dietetics* (New York: John Wiley & Sons, 1977), 49.

2. Ibid., 46.

3. James Trager, *Food Book* (New York: Grossman Publishers, 1970), 262–263.

4. Thomas Jefferson letter to Dr. Vine Utley, March 21, 1819, The Thomas Jefferson Memorial Foundation, Monticello, Charlottesville, Va.

5. Margaret A. Ohlson, "The Philosophy of Dietary Counseling," *Journal of the American Dietetic Association* 63 (1973): 13.

6. Lowell S. Selling and Mary Anna S. Ferraro, *The Psychology of Diet and Nutrition* (New York: W.W. Norton & Company, 1945), 164–166.

7. Ohlson, "Philosophy of Dietary Counseling," 13.

8. Selling and Ferraro, *Psychology of Diet,* 164–166.

9. Buford Stefflre and Kenneth B. Matheny, *The Function of Counseling Theory* (Boston: Houghton Mifflin Company, 1968), 11.

10. Maurice Lorr, "Client Perception of Therapeutic Relation," *Journal of Consulting and Clinical Psychology* 29 (1965): 148.

11. Stefflre and Matheny, *Function of Counseling,* 11.

12. Ibid.

13. Ibid., 12.

14. Carl R. Rogers, *Client-Centered Therapy* (Boston: Houghton Mifflin Company, 1951), 487.

15. John J. Pietrofesa et al., *Counseling: Therapy Research and Practice* (Chicago: Rand McNally College Publishing Company, 1978), 71–72.

16. Albert Ellis, *Reason and Emotion in Psychotherapy* (New York: Lyle Stuart, 1962), 49.

17. Ibid., 28.

18. Pietrofesa et al., *Counseling,* 77.

19. Janet T. Spence et al., *Behavioral Approaches to Therapy* (Morristown, N.J.: General Learning Press, 1976), 5.

20. Pietrofesa et al., *Counseling,* 80–84.

21. Stefflre and Matheny, *Function of Counseling,* 37.

22. Karen Glanz, "Dietitians' Effectiveness and Patient Compliance with Dietary Regimens," *Journal of the American Dietetic Association* 75 (1979): 631.

23. Ibid.

24. Maxine Hosking, "Eating Out: Salt and Hypertension," *The Medical Journal of Australia* 2 (1979): 352.

25. Evan Charney, "Patient-Doctor Communication: Implications for the Clinician," *Pediatric Clinics of North America* 19 (1972): 263.

26. Milton S. Davis, "Variations in Patients' Compliance with Doctors' Orders: Analysis of Congruence between Survey Responses and Results of Empirical Investigations," *Journal of Medical Education* 41 (1966): 1037.

27. Vida Francis, Barbara M. Korsch, and Marie J. Morris, "Gaps in Doctor-Patient Communication: Patients' Responses to Medical Advice," *New England Journal of Medicine* 280 (1969): 535.

28. Barbara S. Hulka et al., "Communication, Compliance, and Concordance between Physician and Patient with Prescribed Medications," *American Journal of Public Health* 66 (1976): 847.

29. Barbara M. Korsch and Vida F. Negrete, "Doctor-Patient Communication," *Scientific American* 227 (1972): 66.

30. Glanz, "Dietitians' Effectiveness," 631.

31. Mason, Wenberg, and Welsch, *Dynamics of Clinical Dietetics,* 65.

32. Norman R. Stewart et al., *Systematic Counseling* (Englewood Cliffs, N.J.: Prentice-Hall, Inc., 1978), 54.

33. Mason, Wenberg, and Welsch, *Dynamics of Clinical Dietetics,* 116.

34. Ibid., 132–134.

35. Ibid., 118.

36. William H. Cormier and L. Sherilyn Cormier, *Interviewing Strategies for Helpers: A Guide to Assessment, Treatment and Evaluation* (Monterey, Calif.: Brooks/Cole Publishing Company, 1979), 183.

37. Ibid., 251.

38. Michael J. Mahoney and Kathryn Mahoney, *Permanent Weight Control, a Solution to the Dieter's Dilemma* (New York: W.W. Norton & Company, 1976), 46–68.

39. Michael J. Mahoney, *Self-Change, Strategies for Solving Personal Problems* (New York: W.W. Norton & Company, 1979), 85–101.

Interviewing Skills

Objectives for Chapter 2

1. List three characteristics necessary in performing optimum nutrition counseling.
2. Define the following three forms of nonverbal behavior: (a) kinesics, (b) paralinguistics, and (c) proxemics.
3. Apply appropriate responses to given client nonverbal behaviors.
4. Apply appropriate listening responses to given client statements.
5. Apply appropriate action responses to given client statements.
6. Apply appropriate sharing responses to given client statements.
7. Apply appropriate teaching responses to given client statements.

2

EFFECTIVE COUNSELOR-CLIENT RELATIONSHIPS

Interviewing skills form the foundation for nutrition counseling (Figure 2–1). To learn interviewing skills, practitioners start, not by examining their clientele, but rather by looking at themselves. What characteristics should an effective nutrition counselor possess?

Personal Characteristics of Counselors

Cormier and Cormier suggest a variety of personal characteristics.[1] Practitioners recognize intuitively that being understanding, conveying respect, and being themselves helps create and maintain a more positively channeled session. The way in which they view themselves and their priorities, values, and expectations can alter the process in a positive or negative way.

Cormier and Cormier focus on three problems with self-image that can result in negative consequences during an interview: competence, power, and intimacy.[2] Individuals' attitudes can involve the concept of competency. Feelings of incompetence can lead to avoidance of controversial issues in counseling sessions. Nutrition counselors may be afraid to say there are no direct or absolute answers to client questions. Providing a truthful answer such as, "The evidence is not in at this time," may be regarded by either the counselors or the clients as evidence of incompetency, the very trait the practitioners hope to avoid.

Closely tied to feelings of incompetence are those of inadequacy, fear of failure, and fear of success. Counselors experiencing these feelings unconsciously tend to try to keep their negative self-images alive by using several behaviors. They may avoid positive interactions by negating positive feedback and making self-deprecating or apologetic comments. For ex-

Figure 2–1 Interviewing Skills As a Foundation for Counseling

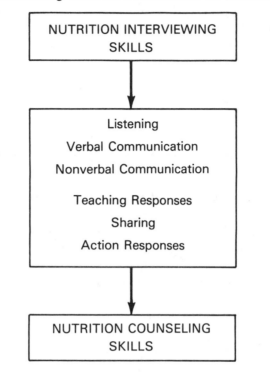

ample, an obese client who has lost weight says, "I really think you're a terrific counselor." A fearful counselor will reply, "Oh, no, I haven't done that much" instead of simply thanking the client for the compliment.

The second potential self-image problem—power—makes counselors feel both omnipotent and fearful of losing control or being weak or unresourceful. In the authoritarian role, counselors try to persuade the clients to obey suggestions without question; practitioners dominate the content and direction of the interview, thinking, "I am in charge." If clients resist or do not respond, the outcome for counselors is resentment and anger. Where weak and unresourceful counselors may occupy a subordinate role, complaining, "If you would just do as I say," the powerful practitioner tends to be dictatorial and overly silent, rarely participates in the interview, and, because of this "I am mightier than thou" attitude, often loses credibility.

The third potential self-image problem focuses on feelings about intimacy. These can involve two extremes—affection and rejection. Counselors who are fearful of rejection will try to elicit only positive feelings from the clients, avoiding confrontation at all costs and ignoring negative cues. This type may even get involved in doing clients favors. Counselors who try to do everything for their clients may be eliminating independent problem solving. Practitioners at the opposite end of the spectrum will try to ignore positive client feelings. They tend to act overly gruff and distant to avoid the closeness that they fear. This type will always try to maintain the authoritarian role of "expert" to maintain distance. (Appendix A presents a counselor self-image checklist.)

How can practitioners determine whether their personal characteristics are conducive to effective counseling? Brammer stresses the importance of being able to answer these two questions: " 'Who am I?' and 'What is important to me?' "[3]

Other authors comment on some of the answers to these questions that may lead to more effective interviews. Loughary and Ripley cite warmth, honesty, sincerity, acceptance, self-confidence, openness, etc., as positive characteristics.[4]

Combs et al. emphasize the importance of counselors' ability to perceive from an internal rather than an external reference point.[5] Those who perceive things internally see themselves as being in control of situations, those who perceive things externally see others as being in charge of the situations. Combs et al. also stress the importance of looking at the world in terms of people rather than things. They describe as good counselors those who see others as able, dependable, friendly, worthy, and helpful and themselves as adequate, worthy, and trustworthy. Such practitioners also view their purposes as altruistic rather than narcissistic and are concerned with larger rather than smaller meanings, being self-revealing rather than self-concealing, involved rather than alienated, and process oriented rather than goal oriented.

Counselors As Growth Facilitators

One of the most crucial of all traits in nutrition counseling is that of facilitating growth—the art of helping clients to achieve their goals and to function on their own. Tyler summarizes successful growth facilitators as accepting, understanding, and sincere (congruence and genuineness).[6] The first step in setting the stage for assuming this role is to show empathy. Brammer states: "The helper sees the world the way the helpee perceives it, that is, from their internal reference."[7] Counselors begin to see the world through their clients' eyes. To facilitate growth, they must be able to provide concrete and specific strategies for behavior change. (See the segments on strategies in Chapter 3, Counseling Skills.)

Facilitative Levels

Researchers have delineated growth facilitative levels that counselors assume at various points in acquiring nutrition interviewing skills.[8,9] The levels listed next illustrate a gradual progression toward a facilitative style— counselors' ability to respond appropriately to clients' problems.

Level 1: The response shows no understanding and no direction in relation to the clients' position. When they bring up a crucial personal topic the counselors start talking about their own personal problems.

Level 2: The response shows no understanding but some direction. The counselors present only general advice: when clients express difficulty with a weight-loss strategy, the response is, "Well, don't worry about it."

Level 3: The response shows understanding but no direction. Counselors might say, "You feel afraid because you're not sure how to avoid food offers from friends."

Level 4: The response shows understanding and some direction. Counselors react to clients' deficits and proposed way of eliminating them by saying, "You feel afraid because you can't say 'no' and you want to avoid eating high-calorie foods."

Level 5: The response shows understanding and specific direction. It contains the deficit, the goal, and one explicit step for overcoming the problem and reaching the objective: "You feel afraid because you can't say 'no' and you want to avoid eating high-calorie foods. One step is to talk with friends about your attempts to lose weight. Elicit their help."

It is important to emphasize that there are no supercounselors who have all of the perfect characteristics to make all sessions successful. Even positive characteristics may not always enhance the interview.

Beyond personal characteristics that affect the sessions are the skills that require practice in development. When these skills are mastered, counseling takes on the characteristics necessary to achieve behavior change.

NONVERBAL COMMUNICATION

Clients' nonverbal behavior can affect the direction of the interview. Effective counselors can use nonverbal cues as signals for unspoken feelings.[10]

Client Nonverbal Behavior

Cormier and Cormier describe three forms of client nonverbal behavior: kinesic, paralinguistic, and proxemic (Exhibit 2–1). Kinesics include a variety of physical behaviors. Paralinguistics refers to how the client's message is delivered. Proxemics involve environmental and personal space.

Exhibit 2–1 presents possible meanings associated with each behavior for each region of the body and a general category of autonomic responses. The developers of this listing (which was designed to cover diet therapy as well as psychological counseling) caution that the effect or meaning of each nonverbal behavior will vary from person to person and culture to culture. The exhibit is designed to increase awareness of different behaviors; it is not intended to make all nutrition counselors experts on all client feelings by using an inventory to generalize meanings applicable to all such individuals. Interpretation of client nonverbal behavior must consider its antecedents and the counselors' responses following the conduct.

The Counselors' Response

Passons describes several ways of responding to nonverbal client behaviors "involving congruence, mixed messages, silence, changing cues, and refocusing for direction."[11] Nutrition counselors can use these suggestions to help in deciding upon a reply.

Congruence

Are the clients' nonverbal messages congruent with the verbal ones? An example might be the individual who comes for the first follow-up weight-loss interview. With furrowed brow, the client sends this confused message to the counselor: "How do I fill in this record? I have forgotten your directions." The counselor can make a mental note of the congruence in behaviors or ask the client to explain the meaning of the nonverbal conduct: "I noticed that your brow was furrowed. What does that mean?" The response could provide information on specifically why the record was not completed. Was it too difficult? Did measuring the foods interfere with meal preparation for the family? Was the counselor's description of the information needed on the record unclear?

Mixed Messages

Is there a mixed message or discrepancy between the verbal and nonverbal messages? For example, a client comes in after having followed a no-added-salt eating pattern for several weeks and states, "It's going really

Exhibit 2–1 Client Nonverbal Behavior Checklist

Nonverbal Dimensions	Behaviors	Description of Counselor-Client Interaction	Possible Effects or Meanings
Kinesics *Eyes*			
_____	Direct eye contact	Client has just shared concern with counselor. Counselor responds; client maintains eye contact.	Readiness or willingness for interpersonal communication or exchange; attentiveness
_____	Lack of sustained eye contact	Each time counselor brings up the topic of client's family, client looks away.	Withdrawal or avoidance of interpersonal exchange; or respect or deference
		Client demonstrates intermittent breaks in eye contact while conversing with counselor.	Respect or deference
		Client mentions sexual concerns, then abruptly looks away. When counselor initiates this topic, client looks away again.	Withdrawal from topic of conversation; discomfort or embarrassment; or preoccupation
_____	Lowering eyes—looking down or away	Client talks at some length about alternatives to present job situation. Pauses briefly and looks down. Then resumes speaking and eye contact with counselor.	Preoccupation
_____	Staring or fixation on person or object	Counselor has just asked client to consider consequences of a certain decision. Client is silent and gazes at a picture on the wall.	Preoccupation; possibly rigidness or uptightness; pondering; difficulty in finding an answer
_____	Darting eyes or blinking rapidly—rapid eye movements; twitching brow	Client indicates desire to discuss a topic yet is hesitant. As counselor probes, client's eyes move around the room rapidly.	Excitation or anxiety; or wearing contact lenses
_____	Squinting or furrow on brow	Client has just asked counselor for advice. Counselor explains role and client squints, and furrows appear in client's brow.	Thought or perplexity; or avoidance of person or topic

Exhibit 2–1 continued

Eyes (cont'd)		Counselor suggests possible things for client to explore in difficulties with parents. Client doesn't respond verbally; furrow in brow appears.	Avoidance of person or topic
_____	Moisture or tears	Client has just reported recent death of father; tears well up in client's eyes.	Sadness; frustration: sensitive areas of concern
		Client reports real progress during past week in marital communication; eyes get moist.	Happiness
_____	Eye shifts	Counselor has just asked client to remember significant events in week; client pauses and looks away; then responds and looks back.	Processing or recalling material; or keen interest; satisfaction
_____	Pupil dilation	Client discusses spouse's sudden disinterest and pupils dilate.	Alarm; or keen interest
		Client leans forward while counselor talks and pupils dilate.	Keen interest; satisfaction
Mouth _____	Smiles	Counselor has just asked client to report positive events of the week. Client smiles, then recounts some of these instances.	Positive thought, feeling, or action in content of conversation; or greeting
		Client responds with a smile to counselor's verbal greeting at beginning of interview.	Greeting
_____	Tight lips (pursed together)	Client has just described efforts at sticking to a difficult living arrangement. Pauses and purses lips together.	Stress or determination; anger or hostility
		Client has just expressed irritation at counselor's lateness. Client sits with lips pursed together while counselor explains the reasons.	Anger or hostility

Exhibit 2–1 continued

Mouth
(cont'd)

	Lower lip quivers or biting of lip	Client starts to describe her recent experience of being raped. As client continues to talk, her lower lip quivers; occasionally she bites her lip.	Anxiety, sadness, or fear
		Client discusses loss of parental support after a recent divorce. Client bites her lip after discussing this.	Sadness
	Open mouth without speaking	Counselor has just expressed feelings about a block in the relationship. Client's mouth drops open; client says was not aware of it.	Surprise; or suppression of yawn—fatigue
		It has been a long session. As counselor talks, client's mouth parts slightly.	Suppression of yawn—fatigue

Facial Expressions

	Eye contact with smiles	Client talks very easily and smoothly, occasionally smiling; maintains eye contact for most of session.	Happiness or comfortableness
	Eyes strained; furrow on brow; mouth tight	Client has just reported strained situation with a child. Client then sits with lips pursed together and frowns.	Anger; or concern; sadness
	Eyes rigid, mouth rigid (unanimated)	Client states: "I have nothing to say"; there is no evident expression or alertness on client's face.	Preoccupation; anxiety; fear

Head

	Nodding head up and down	Client has just expressed concern over own health status; counselor reflects clients' feelings. Client nods head and says "That's right."	Confirmation; agreement; or listening, attending
		Client nods head during counselor explanation.	Listening; attending

Exhibit 2–1 continued

Head (cont'd)			
_____	Shaking head from left to right	Counselor has just suggested that client's continual lateness to sessions may be an issue that needs to be discussed. Client responds with "No," and shakes head from left to right.	Disagreement; or disapproval
_____	Hanging head down, jaw down toward chest	Counselor initiates topic of termination. Client lowers head toward chest, then says "I am not ready to stop the counseling sessions."	Sadness; concern
Shoulders			
_____	Shrugging	Client reports that spouse just walked out with no explanation. Client shrugs shoulders while describing this.	Uncertainty; or ambivalence
_____	Leaning forward	Client has been sitting back in the chair. Counselor discloses something personal; client leans forward and asks counselor a question about the experience.	Eagerness; attentiveness; openness to communication
_____	Slouched, stooped, rounded or turned away from person	Client reports feeling inadequate and defeated because of poor grades; slouches in chair after saying this.	Sadness or ambivalence; or lack of receptivity to interpersonal exchange
		Client reports difficulty in talking. As counselor pursues this, client slouches in chair and turns shoulders away from counselor.	Lack of receptivity to interpersonal exchange
Arms and Hands			
_____	Arms folded across chest	Counselor has just initiated conversation. Client doesn't respond verbally; sits back in chair with arms crossed against chest.	Avoidance of interpersonal exchange; or dislike

Exhibit 2–1 continued

Arms and Hands (cont'd)			
———	Trembling and fidgety hands	Client expresses fear of suicide; hands tremble while talking about this.	Anxiety or anger
		In a loud voice, client expresses resentment; client's hands shake while talking.	Anger
———	Fist clenching of objects or holding hands tightly	Client has just come in for initial interview. Says that he or she feels uncomfortable; hands are clasped together tightly.	Anxiety or anger
		Client expresses hostility toward boss; clenches fists while talking.	Anger
———	Arms unfolded—arms and hands gesturing in conversation	Counselor has just asked a question; client replies and gestures during reply.	Accenting or emphasizing point in conversation; or openness to interpersonal exchange
		Counselor initiates new topic. Client readily responds; arms are unfolded at this time.	Openness to interpersonal exchange
———	Rarely gesturing, hands and arms stiff	Client arrives for initial session. Responds to counselor's questions with short answers. Arms are kept down at side.	Tension or anger
		Client has been referred; sits with arms down at side while explaining reasons for referral and irritation at being here.	Anger
Legs and Feet			
———	Legs and feet appear comfortable and relaxed	Client's legs and feet are relaxed without excessive movement while client freely discusses personal concerns.	Openness to interpersonal exchange; relaxation
———	Crossing and uncrossing legs repeatedly	Client is talking rapidly in spurts about problems; continually crosses and uncrosses legs while doing so.	Anxiety; depression

Exhibit 2–1 continued

Legs and Feet (cont'd)			
_____	Foot-tapping	Client is tapping feet during a lengthy counselor summary; client interrupts counselor to make a point.	Anxiety; impatience—wanting to make a point
_____	Legs and feet appear stiff and controlled	Client is open and relaxed while talking about job. When counselor introduces topic of marriage, client's legs become more rigid.	Uptightness or anxiety; closed to extensive interpersonal exchange
Total Body			
_____	Facing other person squarely or leaning forward	Client shares a concern and faces counselor directly while talking; continues to face counselor while counselor responds.	Openness to interpersonal communication and exchange
_____	Turning of body orientation at an angle, not directly facing person, or slouching in seat	Client indicates some difficulty in "getting into" interview. Counselor probes for reasons; client turns body away.	Less openness to interpersonal exchange
_____	Rocking back and forth in chair or squirming in seat	Client indicates a lot of nervousness about an approaching conflict situation. Client rocks as this is discussed.	Concern; worry; anxiety
_____	Stiff—sitting erect and rigidly on edge of chair	Client indicates some uncertainty about direction of interview; sits very stiff and erect.	Tension; anxiety; concern

Paralinguistics

Voice Level and Pitch

_____	Whispering or inaudibility	Client has been silent for a long time. Counselor probes; client responds, but in a barely audible voice.	Difficulty in disclosing
_____	Pitch changes	Client is speaking at a moderate voice level while discussing job. Then client begins to talk about boss and voice pitch rises considerably.	Topics of conversation have different emotional meanings

Exhibit 2–1 continued

Fluency in Speech			
_____	Stuttering, hesitations, speech errors	Client is talking rapidly about feeling uptight in certain social situations; client stutters and makes some speech errors while doing so.	Sensitivity about topic in conversation; or anxiety and discomfort
_____	Whining or lisp	Client is complaining about having a hard time losing weight; voice goes up like a whine.	Dependency or emotional emphasis
_____	Rate of speech slow, rapid, or jerky	Client begins interview talking slowly about a bad weekend. As topic shifts to client's feelings about self, client talks more rapidly.	Sensitivity to topics of conversation; or topics have different emotional meanings
_____	Silence	Client comes in and counselor invites client to talk; client remains silent.	Reluctance to talk; or preoccupation
		Counselor has just asked client a question. Client pauses and thinks over a response.	Preoccupation; or desire to continue speaking after making a point; thinking about how to respond
		A Chinese client talks about own family. Pauses; then resumes conversation to talk more about same subject.	Desire to continue speaking after making a point
Autonomic Responses			
_____	Clammy hands, shallow breathing, sweating, pupil dilation, paleness, blushing, rashes on neck	Client discusses the exciting prospect of having two desirable job offers. Breathing becomes faster and client's pupils dilate.	Arousal—positive (excitement, interest) or negative (anxiety, embarrassment)
		Client starts to discuss sexual concerns; breathing becomes shallow and red splotches appear on neck.	Anxiety, embarrassment

Exhibit 2–1 continued

Proxemics
Distance

_____	Moves away	Counselor has just confronted client; client moves back before responding verbally.	Signal that space has been invaded; increased arousal, discomfort
_____	Moves closer	Midway through session, client moves chair toward helper.	Seeking closer interaction, more intimacy

Position in Room

_____	Sits behind or next to an object in the room, such as table or desk	A new client comes in and sits in a chair that is distant from counselor.	Seeking protection or more space
_____	Sits near counselor without any intervening objects	A client who has been in to see counselor before sits in chair closest to counselor.	Expression of adequate comfort level

Source: Adapted from *Interviewing Strategies for Helpers* by William H. Cormier and L. Sherilyn Cormier, published by Brooks/Cole Publishing Company, Monterey, Calif., pp. 32–38. Copyright © 1979, by permission of Brooks/Cole Publishing Company.

[pause] well. I've had [pause] very few problems," while looking down and leaning away. The nutrition counselor can deal with these discrepancies in one of three ways: (1) to just take mental note; (2) to describe the discrepancy to the client, for example, "You say the diet is really going well and that there are few problems but you were looking down and really spoke with a lot of hesitation "; (3) to reply, "I noticed you looked away and paused as you said that. What does that mean?"

Silence

Are there nonverbal behaviors with silence? Silence does not mean that nothing is happening. It can have different meanings from one culture to another.[12]

In some cultures silence denotes respect.[13] Sue and Sue point out that for the Chinese and Japanese, silence means a desire to resume speaking after making a point. Once again the nutrition counselor can mentally note the silence, describe it to the client or ask the person to explain it.

Changing Cues

Is it necessary to distract or interrupt clients by focusing on nonverbal behavior? This may be needed to change the flow of the interview because continuation of the topic may be unproductive. If clients are pouring out a lot of information or are rambling, a change in the direction of the interview may be useful. In such instances, nutrition counselors can distract the clients from the verbal content by refocusing on nonverbal behavior.

For example, for unproductive content in a client's messages, a counselor might say, "Our conversation so far has been dealing with your inability to cope with your spouse's unsupportive comments about your weight-control diet. Are you aware that you have been gripping the sides of your chair with your hands while you speak?"

Nutrition counselors must decide very carefully whether or not such distractions can be destructive or productive to the interview. If the change in flow makes the clients feel unable to continue to air feelings, the distraction could be detrimental. Experienced counselors probably will find that their own intuition helps in knowing when to interrupt.

Refocusing for Redirection

Are there pronounced changes in the clients' nonverbal behavior? Initially they may sit with arms crossed, then become more relaxed, with arms unfolded and hands gesturing. Once again counselors can respond either overtly or covertly.

Counselor Nonverbal Communication

The counselors' nonverbal communication can have a great impact on the relationship. Based on analogue research, Cormier and Cormier report that the nonverbal counselor behaviors that seem to be most important include expressions in the eyes and face, head nodding and smiles, body orientation and posture, some vocal cues, and physical distance between practitioners and clients.[14] To help counselors determine whether or not they are demonstrating desirable behaviors, they can ask someone to observe their nonverbal behaviors. Appendix B is a checklist a third-party observer can mark while evaluating the counselor's nonverbal behavior. One word of caution: counselors should not try to apply these behaviors to themselves in a rigid way. Inflexible conformity can increase their tension in an interview and their nonverbal expression of that tension will be sensed and increased by clients.

VERBAL COMMUNICATION

The counselors' knowledge and command of verbal skills can play an important part in directing the interview.

Conversational Style

Beginning counselors tend to fall into a kind of conversational mode that is very comfortable for them. Such a style is typical of a friendly chat with a neighbor. A second common pitfall is the extreme pressure they feel in trying to provide a solution for the client's problem.

There are certain aspects of conversational style that interfere with the objectives of counseling:[15]

1. Cocktail party "small talk": Responding to a client at the beginning of an interview with, "Did you see the diet recipes in today's paper?"
2. Expressions of blame, criticism, or judgments: Client: "The diet has gone badly this week." Nutrition Counselor: "I can certainly see that from this weight graph."
3. Expressions of advice offered in a preaching or self-righteous tone: "You should really learn to have more self-control with this diet," or "You really ought to lose 20 pounds."
4. Expressions of sympathy in a patronizing tone: "I really feel sorry for you. You seem to get absolutely no support from your family in following this diet," or "Now that you've told me your problems with weight loss, I'm sure I can make you feel better."
5. Threats or arguing: "You'd better follow the low-calorie diet for your own good," or "I think your constant rejection of my suggestions is uncalled for."
6. Rigidity or inflexibility: "There is only one right way to approach weight loss," or "Your suggestions won't work with a low-sodium diet."
7. Overanalyzing, overinterpreting, or intellectualizing: "I think you find being overweight enjoyable or otherwise you would follow the diet."
8. Several questions at once: "How do you feel about following a low-cholesterol diet? Does it fit into your family life? If 'no,' why isn't it working out? Could you tell me?"
9. Extensive self-disclosure, sharing the counselor's own problems: "I've been thinking a lot about my weight loss attempts as you were talking. I, too, have had several problems. For instance . . ."

Counselor-Client Focus Identification

Once the conversational style has been altered appropriately, there are several specific ways in which nutrition counselors can learn to provide direction and focus for an interview. Six categories of subject focus and three areas of verbal focus can be stated in past, present, or future time.

The six categories of subject focus are delineated by Ivey and Gluckstern:

1. Client focused (subject is "you")
2. Counselor focused (subject is "I")
3. Others focused (subject is "they")
4. Relationship of group focused (subject is "we")
5. Topic focused (subject is a noun, such as diet, sodium, calories, etc.)
6. Culture-environment focused (subject is society, culture, or environment. For example the counselor might say, "Society today seems to idealize thinness.")[16]

Lavelle and Cormier suggest three areas of focus indicated by the verb in the sentence:

1. affective focused
2. behavioral focused
3. cognitive focused.[17,18]

The verb "to feel" is used frequently when counselors want to focus affectively: "You are feeling very frustrated by your desire to follow the diet and your family's uncooperativeness." Behavioral focused sentences usually contain verbs such as "to do," "to act," or "to behave," as in, "What are you doing about this?" A cognitive focus is revealed by such verbs as "to think" or "to tell oneself": "What are you telling yourself when you eat the entire pie?"

The verb can be in the past, present, or future tense, which determines the time focus of the sentence. Too much focus on the past or future may indicate an avoidance of the present. An example might be this description of weight loss by one client:

"My first husband was always supportive. My second husband wants me to be small but he always tempts me with high-calorie snacks. Still, he always talks about the future when I will be thin."

This client is dwelling on both the past and the future but does not seem to recognize the importance of present goal setting.

The following examples show how verbal focusing might be used in response to a client who says: "I'm having a conflict about wanting to lose weight but have no one at home who supports me when we eat out."

1. Client-Cognitive—Present Focus: "You find yourself thinking about wanting to lose weight but also wanting to eat out with the family." In this response, the client-subject focus is reflected in "You find yourself," the cognitive focus by "thinking about," and the present time focus by the present tense of the verb "find."
2. Client-Affective—Present Focus: "You're feeling concerned about wanting to lose weight and also wanting to eat out with your family."
3. Group-Behavioral—Future Focus: "Perhaps this is an area we will explore together and see what you can do."
4. Topic-Cognitive—Present Focus: "Losing weight is not always easy. When I think about it, there are lots of obstacles to try to overcome."
5. Cultural/Environmental-Cognitive/Behavioral—Past Focus: "This is a conflict many weight loss clients have faced because of the ideas our culture has given us about what people should eat in social situations."

LISTENING RESPONSES

Listening responses are the first step in forming a repertoire of counseling skills involving:

1. clarification
2. paraphrase
3. reflection
4. summarization.

Clarification

Clarification is posing a question, often after an ambiguous client message. Clarification may be used to make the previous message explicit and to confirm the accuracy of the counselors' perceptions of it. An example of incorrect use of clarification is:

CLIENT: "I wish I didn't have to fill in those diet records. They seem so silly to me."
COUNSELOR: "Why don't you like my diet aids?"

CLIENT: "I like all of them and the record has been useful but I just don't feel as though it is helping me at this point."

In the next example, a statement of clarification establishes exactly what was said without relying on assumptions and inferences that are not confirmed or explored:

CLIENT: "I wish I didn't have to fill in those diet records. They seem so silly to me."
COUNSELOR: "Are you saying that you don't see any purpose to filling in the diet record?"
CLIENT: "No, I really don't. I just don't think I need them at this point."

Paraphrase

Paraphrase is a restatement or rephrasing of the clients' message in the counselors' own words. For example, the client says: "I don't mind following the diet at home but my job requires that I travel one week of every month. It is impossible to follow the diet when eating in restaurants!" In paraphrasing, counselors can:

1. restate the message to themselves
2. identify the content part of the message ("I don't mind following the diet at home," "My job requires one week of travel a month," "It is impossible to follow the diet when eating in restaurants.")
3. translate the message into their own words. ("You can follow the diet at home but have problems following it in restaurants.")

Reflection

Reflection of feelings is used to rephrase the affective part of the message. This form of listening response has three purposes:

1. to encourage expression of more feelings
2. to help clients experience feelings more intensely so they can become aware of unresolved problems
3. to help clients become more aware of feelings that dominate them.

For example, a client comments: "I feel so depressed. Sometimes dieting seems useless." In reply, counselors can:

1. restate the client's message covertly
2. identify the affective part of the message ("I feel so depressed")
3. translate the clients' affect words into their own words. ("You sometimes feel frustrated with dieting.")

One word of caution: a reflection is more than just beginning a statement with the words "You feel . . . ." It is a reflecting back of the emotional part of the message with appropriate affect words. (Commonly used affect words are listed in Exhibit 2–2.)

Summarization

The fourth listening response is summarization. This requires extending the paraphrase and reflection responses. It is a rather complex skill that includes paying attention to both content and feelings. It also includes elements of purpose, timing, and effect of the statements (process). In these guidelines for summarization, Brammer recommends that counselors:

1. Attend to major topics and emotions apparent as the client speaks.
2. Summarize key ideas into broad statements.

Exhibit 2–2 List of Commonly Used Affect Words

Happiness	Sadness	Fear	Uncertainty	Anger
Happy	Discouraged	Scared	Puzzled	Upset
Pleased	Disappointed	Anxious	Confused	Frustrated
Satisfied	Hurt	Frightened	Unsure	Bothered
Glad	Despairing	Defensive	Uncertain	Annoyed
Optimistic	Depressed	Threatened	Skeptical	Irritated
Good	Disillusioned	Afraid	Doubtful	Resentful
Relaxed	Dismayed	Tense	Undecided	Mad
Content	Pessimistic	Nervous	Bewildered	Outraged
Cheerful	Miserable	Uptight	Mistrustful	Hassled
Thrilled	Unhappy	Uneasy	Insecure	Offended
Delighted	Hopeless	Worried	Bothered	Angry
Excited	Lonely	Panicked	Disoriented	Furious

Source: Reprinted from *Interviewing Strategies for Helpers* by William H. Cormier and L. Sherilyn Cormier, with permission of Brooks/Cole Publishing Company, © 1979, p. 69.

3. Do not add new ideas.
4. Decide whether it is wise for you as a counselor to summarize or ask the client to summarize the broad themes, agreements, or plans.

To make this decision, [counselors should] review the purpose of the summarization:

1. Was it to encourage the client at the beginning of the interview?
2. Was it to bring scattered thoughts and feelings into focus?
3. Was it to close the discussion on the major theme of the interview?
4. Was it to check your understanding of the interview's progress?
5. Was it to encourage the client to explore the basic theme of the interview more carefully?
6. Was it to end the relationship with a progress summary?
7. Was it to reassure the client that the interview was progressing well?[19]

Many summarization responses include references to both cognitive and affective messages:

CLIENT: "I want to follow the diet we discussed but so many things pull me toward food—parties, friends, my family, etc. Above all this, though, I know I want to lose weight."
COUNSELOR: "You feel torn. You want to lose weight but sometimes you feel reluctant to avoid all of the people and things pulling you toward food" (summarization of emotion) or "You know that you do want to lose weight" (summarization of contents).

ACTION RESPONSES

These listening responses deal primarily with the clients' message from their point of view. It is essential to the progress of the nutrition counseling process to move beyond the clients' point of view to use of responses based on counselor-generated data and perceptions. These are counselor directed and are labeled active responses. They involve a combination of the following:

1. counselor perceptions
2. counselor hypotheses

3. client messages
4. client behaviors.[20]

The purpose of active responses is to help clients recognize the need for change and positive action in solving nutrition problems. Active replies include:

1. probing responses
2. attributing responses
3. confronting responses
4. interpreting responses.[21]

Probing

In nutrition counseling, a most important part of gathering information on clients' eating patterns involves the art of probing. Probing can involve both open and closed questions. Initially, probing should be aimed at eliciting the most information possible. The clients should feel free to respond at length to any problem that may limit adherence to the eating pattern. The most direct way of achieving this purpose is to ask open-ended questions. These begin with "what," "when," "how," "where," "why," or "who." Such questions require more than just "yes" or "no" responses. Their purposes can be varied:

1. to begin an interview
2. to encourage client elaboration or to obtain information
3. to elicit specific examples of client's nutrition-related behaviors, feelings, or thoughts
4. to ask for expressions of feeling from the client.[22]

Once the clients have provided information adequate for assessment of the nutrition problem, counselors can help focus attention on central issues by using closed questions.[23] When the clients then have a focus on which to concentrate, open invitations to talk may be used again. In becoming skilled interviewers, the counselors will learn to use a balance of open and closed questions. Various types of interviews use different proportions of open and closed questions.

An example of the use of probes: The client (a 25-year-old male who is trying to follow a 300-milligram cholesterol diet) complains: "I really have problems getting my wife to cook low-cholesterol meals. She says she wants to cook the way her mother taught her. I feel really frustrated about everything."

The counselor responds with open-ended probes:

- "What else do you think or feel frustrated about?"
- "How long have you been feeling this way?"
- "When are some specific times you feel frustrated?"
- "Who are you with when you feel frustrated?"
- "What do you do when you feel frustrated?"

After the client has discussed at length several specific frustrating instances, the counselor can focus the interview with closed probes such as:

- "Is your wife aware that you feel frustrated in these situations?"
- "Have you spoken to your wife about these frustrating instances?"
- "Can you speak with your wife about these problem situations?"
- "Do you see any solutions to this particular frustration?"

Attributing

Attributing responses point to the clients' current potential for being successful in a designated activity. This response has several purposes:

1. to encourage the client who lacks initiative or self-confidence to do something
2. to expand the client's awareness of personal strength
3. to point out a potentially helpful client action.[24]

It is important in deciding whether or not to use this response to focus on inferring how the clients will react. Will the attributing response "reinforce the client's action-seeking behavior or the client's feelings of inadequacy?"[25] This response should be used only when there is a basis for recognizing the clients' ability to pursue desired action. It should not be used simply as a pep talk to smooth over or discount their true feelings of discouragement. Feelings should be reflected and clarified first. Finally, the ability or attributing response should be used when they are ready for action but seem hesitant to jump in or initiate a step without some prior encouragement.

An example of an ability response:

CLIENT (a 30-year-old woman who has tried repeatedly to lose weight): "I'm really discouraged with trying to lose weight at this point. I feel like I can't do anything right. Not only has it affected me personally but now it is affecting my family. I just don't feel like I can do anything right."

COUNSELOR: "Although you feel discouraged with weight loss right now, you still have those personal qualities you had when you lost weight before."

Confronting

A confronting response can be a descriptive statement of clients' mixed messages or an identification of an alternate view or perception of something the individuals distort. There are two intended purposes behind a confronting response:

1. to identify the client's mixed or distorted messages
2. to explore other ways of perceiving the client's self or situation.[26]

Confronting responses can have very powerful effects. There are several basic rules that should be kept in mind before using them. Counselors should:

1. Make the confronting response a description instead of a judgment or evaluation of the client's message or behavior.
2. Cite specific examples of the behavior rather than making vague inferences.
3. Prior to confronting the client, build rapport and trust.
4. Offer the confrontation when the client is most likely to accept it.
5. Do not overload the client with confrontations that make heavy demands in a short time.[27]

It is important to keep in mind the timing of a confronting response. A confrontation should always take place at a time when clients will not feel threatened, not when it is totally unexpected. Adequate time for talking and listening should be provided in the interview.

The counselors' feelings also are important. Johnson clearly emphasizes confronting the clients only if the practitioners are genuinely interested in improving the relationship,[28] never with the idea of punishing or criticizing the individuals. Before confronting, counselors should try to list their reasons for wanting to challenge discrepancies, distortions, or unproductive behaviors.

Johnson describes eight components of effective confrontation by counselors (Exhibit 2–3).[29]

Exhibit 2–3 Components of Effective Confrontation

1. *Personal statements*: These opening statements usually begin with the pronoun "I." Included in this statement are expressions of feelings, attitudes, or opinions. Examples are:

   "I need to talk to you."

   "There is something I've been hearing over and over in our conversation that I would like to speak to you about."

   "I have been confused during this session by something you've been saying."

2. *Relationship statements*: Defines your relationship with the other person. An example is:

   "Lately we've been trying to work together to come up with some possible solutions to your binge eating."

3. *Description of behavior*: A description of a specific behavior would include specific time and place of occurrence. An example is:

   "From your description, binge eating occurs on weekends during parties."

4. *Descriptions of your feelings and interpretations of the client's situation*: An example:

   "I am confused when you say that you want to stop eating at parties but you feel compelled to continue because of social pressure. There seem to be two messages here."

5. *Understanding response:* This is to be sure that what you have said is what the client has understood.

   COUNSELOR: "Do you see what I mean?" "Is this the way you see things?"

   CLIENT: "Yes."

6. *Perception check:* This is stated as a question to the client to double-check thoughts and feelings at this point.

   COUNSELOR: "How do you feel about what I am saying?"

   CLIENT: "I can see that I seem to be giving a mixed message. I want to lose weight but there are always obstacles when I go to parties. Friends always ask me to eat; I feel compelled to say "Yes."

7. *Interpretive response:* This is a paraphrase of what the client said in 5 and 6:

   "From what you have said, you seem to feel this same confusion. You want to lose weight but there is always someone pushing you to eat to be sociable."

8. *Constructive feedback:* This component of confrontation calls for working together for a solution. Alternatives are presented and weighed. The counselor, at this point, should allow the client to make suggestions on how to solve the problem:

   "Can you think of a solution?"

   "This might be one solution. What else can we come up with?"

   "I'd like to talk about it again after we've thought about it for a while."

Source: Adapted from *Reaching Out: Interpersonal Effectiveness and Self-Actualization* by David W. Johnson, published by Prentice-Hall, Englewood Cliffs, N.J., p. 165. Copyright © 1972, by permission of Prentice-Hall.

The clients' reaction to a confrontation can be varied. Cormier and Cormier describe four types:

1. denial
2. confusion
3. false acceptance
4. genuine acceptance.[30]

Egan lists specific ways clients might deny the confrontation:

1. Discredit the counselor: "How could you know when you've never had the problem of being overweight?"
2. Persuade the counselor that his or her views are wrong or misinterpreting: "I really do want to lose weight. I try very hard. I think this diet you gave me is too high in calories."
3. Devaluate the importance of the topic: "I'm not sure this is worth all of my time. I could just take diet pills."
4. Seek support elsewhere: "I told my husband about your comment and he thinks I must accept friends' offers of food at parties."[31]

If clients seem confused about the meaning of the confrontation, the counselors may not have been specific or concise enough; or, confessed lack of understanding may be a way of avoiding the impact of the confrontation.

Sometimes the clients may seem to accept the confrontation. If the individuals show a sincere desire to change behavior, their acceptance probably is genuine. However, they may agree verbally with the counselors but, instead of pursuing the confrontation, may have done so only to get the practitioners not to discuss the topic in the future.

There is no defined way to deal with negative reactions to a confrontation. But the Johnson components can be used to go back and repeat the relationship statement or describe the counselor's own feelings and perceptions. The sequence might go like this:

COUNSELOR: "Both of our goals are to help eliminate binge eating at parties." (Relationship Statement)

CLIENT: "Actually I'm not sure I can ever achieve that even though I do want to lose weight." (Mixed Message)

COUNSELOR: "You say you want to lose weight but one of the major causes is too difficult to overcome." (Description of Counselor Feelings and Perceptions)

CLIENT: "No, I guess you just don't understand. You've never been in my shoes." (Discredit the Counselor)

COUNSELOR: "Because I've never been in your shoes doesn't mean we can't work on a solution together. I have had experience with many cases like yours. You seem to exhibit many qualities that show me that you can handle this problem." (Attributing Statement) "You are open about the difficulties you face and can describe specific instances where problems occur." (Attributing Statement) "Let's look at those specifics and try to come up with some solutions." (Constructive Feedback)

Interpreting

An interpreting response is an active reply that gives a possible explanation of or association among various client behaviors. It has three intended purposes:

1. to identify the relationship between the clients' behavior and nonverbal and verbal messages
2. to examine the clients' behavior using a variety of views or different explanations
3. to help clients gain self-understanding as a basis for behavior change or action.

There are several specific ground rules.[32] Counselors must be careful about timing. Clients should demonstrate some degree of readiness for self-exploration or self-examination before an interpreting response is used. This is best given at the beginning or middle phase of an interview so both counselors and clients have sufficient time to work through the latter's reaction. It is important to be sure the counselors' interpretation is based on the clients' actual message. Practitioners must eliminate their own biases and values. They must offer the interpretive response tentatively, using such words as, "I wonder if," "It's possible that," "Perhaps," or "Maybe." Clients should be asked whether the message is accurate.

Brammer offers these guidelines for counselors in interpreting responses:

1. Look for the clients' basic messages.
2. Paraphrase these to the clients.
3. Add your own understanding of what their messages mean (motives, defenses, needs, styles, etc.).
4. Keep the language simple and the level close to their [the clients'] message.

5. Indicate that you are offering tentative ideas.
6. Elicit the clients' reactions to your interpretations.[33]

Ivey and Authier describe the interpreting response as a part of the essence of what the clients have said (emotionally and intellectually) and as a summary that adds other relevant data.[34]

The following is an example of an interpreting response:

CLIENT (an overweight middle-aged man): "I'm really discouraged with this dieting. I am at the point where I feel like I can't win. I've been to doctors and weight-loss groups. I've taken diet pills. It's at the point where I can't think straight at work because my thoughts are always on dieting. I feel very depressed."

COUNSELOR: "I wonder if you're allowing your preoccupation with weight loss to interfere with your ability to cope?" (This interpreting response makes an association between the client's desire to lose weight and resulting feelings and behavior.)

Or: "Is it possible that you're trying to find an easy, magic way to lose weight when that solution may not exist?" (This interpreting response offers a possible explanation of the client's weight-loss behaviors.)

SHARING RESPONSES

Counselors can use two sharing responses: self-disclosure and immediacy. The sharing responses involve counselor self-expression and usually contain content that refers to the practitioner, the client, or emotions of either one.

Self-Disclosure

Self-disclosure is a response in which counselors verbally share information about themselves. Cormier and Cormier describe four purposes:

1. to provide an open, facilitative counseling atmosphere
2. to increase the client's perceived similarity between self and the counselor to reduce distance resulting from role differences
3. to provide a model to assist in increasing the client's disclosure level
4. to influence the client's perceived or actual behavioral changes.[35]

There are several basic ideas to keep in mind before using self-disclosure. Counselors who rarely self-disclose may add to the role distance between themselves and their clients. At the other extreme, too much self-disclosure may be counterproductive. The length of time spent in self-disclosing should not be excessively long or short.[36-38] Self-disclosing statements should be similar in content and mood to the clients' message.

Self-disclosure can be of several types:

1. demographic[39]
2. personal[40]
3. positive[41]
4. negative.[42]

In demographic disclosures, counselors talk about nonintimate events:

"I have had some failures in low-cholesterol meal preparation, also."

"I have not always used self-control skills to their optimum in assuring a balanced diet."

In personal disclosures, counselors reveals more private personal events:

"Well, I don't always feel loving toward my husband (wife), especially when he (she) is nonsupportive of my efforts in meal preparation."

"I think it is very natural to want to please close friends. There are times when I've accepted food at parties when I really didn't want it but I cared so much about the person offering it that I couldn't say 'No.' "

In positive self-disclosure, counselors reveal positive strengths, coping skills, or positive successful experiences:

"I'm really a task-oriented person. When I decide what must be done, I work until the task is completed."

"It's important to be as open with my husband (wife) as possible. When he (she) upsets me, I try to tell him (her) honestly exactly how I feel."

In negative self-disclosure, counselors provide information about personal limitations or difficult experiences:

"I also have trouble expressing opinions. I guess I am wishy-washy a lot of the time."

"Sometimes I'm also afraid to tell my husband (wife) how I really feel. Then my frustration builds to a climax and I just explode."

Ivey and Authier list four key dimensions of self-disclosure:

1. the personal pronoun "I"
2. expression of content or feeling
3. object of the sentence (one's own experience)

4. tense of the verb in the statement (past tense is safer for both the counselor and client; however, present tense has more impact and is more powerful).[43]

Two examples of self-disclosure can apply to the same situation: the client is feeling like a failure because no one seems to support the person's weight loss. The counselor responds:

"I, too, have felt down about myself at times."

"I can remember feeling depressed when everyone seemed to take lightly something that was important to me, like eating a favorite dish at my favorite restaurant."

Immediacy

The second sharing response, immediacy, involves counselors' reflections on a present aspect of a thought or feeling about self, clients, or a significant relationship issue. The verbal expression of immediacy may include the listening responses of reflection and summation, the active responses of confrontation and interpretation, and the sharing response of self-disclosure. Examples of the three categories of immediacy are:

1. Counselor immediacy: The counselor reveals personal thoughts of immediacy at the moment they occur: "It's good to see you again;" or "I'm sorry I didn't follow that. I seem to have trouble focusing today. Let's go over that again."
2. Client immediacy: The counselor states something about the client's behavior or feeling as it occurs in the interview: "You seem uncomfortable now;" or "You're really smiling now. You must be very pleased."
3. Relationship immediacy: The counselor reveals personal feelings or thoughts about experiencing the relationship: "I'm glad that you are able to share those feelings you have about following the diet with me;" or "It makes me feel good that we've been able to resolve some of the problems with your diet."

Immediacy has two purposes: (1) This response can be used to bring covert feelings or unresolved relationship issues into the open for discussion. (2) It also can provide immediate feedback about counselor and client feelings and aspects of the relationship as they occur in the session.

When making an immediacy response, counselors should:

1. describe what they see as it happens
2. reflect the "here and nowness" of the experience

3. reserve this response for initiating exploration of the most significant or most influential feelings or issues.

TEACHING RESPONSES

Much of nutrition counselors' work involves teaching clients how to change eating behaviors. Change means that they learn new ways to deal with themselves, others, or environmental situations. The counselors may teach new eating behaviors, new awareness of past and present ones, or new perceptions of past and present ones—or how clients can teach themselves. Three verbal responses associated with teaching and learning can give structure to what ordinarily might be haphazard teaching: instructions, verbal setting operations, and information giving.[44]

Instructions

Instructions involve one or more statements in which the counselors tell the clients what eating behaviors are required, how they might occur, and allowable limits within which to perform them. When using instruction responses, counselors instruct, direct, or cue the clients to do something. Instructions may deal with what should happen within or outside the interview and can be both informing and influential.

Instructions have two main purposes:

1. to influence or give cues to help clients respond in a certain way
2. to provide information necessary to acquire, strengthen, or eliminate a response.

After giving instructions, counselors should check to ascertain whether the clients really understand the directions. Clients are asked to repeat what was said to help the counselors know whether they communicated the message accurately. The counselors then exhort the clients to use the instructions.

Instructions can be worded in many ways. "You should do something" is likely to put a client on the defensive—it is too demanding. More useful words are, "I'd like you to," "I'd appreciate it," or "I think it would help if." Clients are more likely to follow instructions that are linked to positive or rewarding consequences.[45]

Exhibit 2–4 presents examples of information giving both in and outside of a nutrition counseling session.

Exhibit 2–4 Aspects of Information Giving

Counselor's Instructions	In the Interview	Outside the Interview
What to do	"Please repeat what I have asked you to do in responding to your husband's (wife's) nonsupportiveness toward your diet. I want to be sure I am communicating the request accurately."	"Please keep a record of your thoughts before your conversations with your husband (wife)."
How to do	"When you say this, pretend that I am your husband (wife). Look at me and maintain eye contact while you say it."	"Write your thoughts down on a note card and bring them in next week."
Allowable limits	"Say it in a strong, firm voice. Don't speak in a soft, weak voice. Look at me while you say it."	"Remember to record these thoughts before, not after, you speak."

Verbal Setting Operation

The second teaching response, the verbal setting operation, attempts to predispose someone to view a situation or an event in a certain way before it takes place. This response includes a statement describing a treatment and the potential value of counseling and/or treatment for clients. The purposes of verbal setting operations are to motivate clients to understand the purpose of and to use counseling and/or treatment.

Goldstein suggests that some initial counseling structure may prevent negative feelings in clients because they lack information about what to expect.[46] He feels that initial structuring should focus upon and clarify counselor and client role expectations. This type of structuring should be "detailed, deliberate and repeated."[47]

The following are examples of verbal setting operations:

Overview of nutrition counseling: The counselor says: "I believe it would be helpful if I first talked about what nutrition involves. We will spend some time talking together to find out first the kinds of nutrition concerns you have and what you want to do about them. Then we will work as a team to try to meet them. Sometimes I may ask you to do some things on your own outside the session."

Purpose of nutrition counseling: The counselor says: "These sessions may help you change food behaviors to achieve weight loss. The action plans you'll carry out—with my assistance—can help you learn to eat wisely in situations that may be of concern to you."

The persons' understanding of nutrition counseling can be checked by asking, "How does this fit with your expectations?"

Information Giving

Much of the nutrition counselors' responsibility involves the third teaching response—information giving. Cormier and Cormier give specific guidelines to follow when giving information:

1. Identify information presently available to client.
2. Evaluate client's present information. Is it valid? Data-based? Sufficient? Insufficient?

The following guidelines can be used in determining what information to give:

1. Identify the kind of information useful to the client.
2. Identify possible reliable sources of information.
3. Identify any preferred sequencing of information, i.e., option A before option B.

The following guidelines indicate how to deliver information:

1. Limit the amount of information given at one time.
2. Ask for and discuss client's feelings and biases about information.
3. Know when to stop giving information so action isn't avoided.
4. Wait for the client's cue of readiness for additional information after providing a large group of facts.
5. Present all relevant facts; don't protect clients from negative information. [48]

CHOOSING THE APPROPRIATE RESPONSE

One of the most important processes in counseling involves deciding when to use the responses just described. Steps toward determining appropriate responses include (1) identification of the purposes of the interview and of the counselor responses and (2) assessment of the effects of the selected replies and strategies on client answers and outcomes. When one response or strategy does not achieve its intended purpose, the counselors use discrimination to identify and select another that is more likely to achieve the desired results or focus.

Cormier and Cormier describe three parts of an interview that can be used in determining which responses or strategies to select:

1. Counselor identifies purposes of the interview and responses.
2. Counselor selects and implements the response.
3. Counselor determines if resulting client verbal and nonverbal responses achieve the purpose or distract from the purpose.[49]

These authors also describe a step-by-step process for counselors in conducting an effective interview:

1. Define the purpose of the interview.
2. Define the purpose of your initial response.
3. Make your initial response.
4. Identify client verbal and nonverbal responses.
5. Label those client responses as goal related or distracting.
6. Set a plan for the next response.[50]

Nutrition counselors' first step is to listen carefully to each client statement. They must think about whether it is related to or distracts from the purposes of the interview. Once this determination has been made, counselors can select and use responses they believe will achieve the objective. If client responses are goal related, practitioners may decide that their own replies and comments are on target; however, if they note several statements that are distracting, they may need to analyze what they have been saying.

For example, one of the major goals of a counseling session may be to identify steps to help change eating behaviors in an overweight adult male. The counselor has suggested cutting down on midmorning snacking by switching from high-calorie snack foods that are low in nutrients to more low-calorie, high-nutrient foods. The client indicates that this will not work for him. After determining that this is a distracting client response, the practitioner will need to formulate and use an alternate response—perhaps a new action step. Regardless of what that next response is, the important point is that the counselor can identify a purpose or direction, assess whether the resulting client answers are related to that goal, and select alternative replies with a rationale in mind.

Counselors should make these assessments cognitively, i.e., in their heads. This step-by-step procedure should be used in thinking through an interview. What follows is an example of how those steps might apply in a nutrition counseling session.

Interview purpose: To listen to the client (a 26-year-old woman) describe factors contributing to her inability to lose weight over the past two years. (Details of the interview objective and the relationship between client and counselor are not included here.)

1. COUNSELOR: "According to your chart, Dr. B. sent you to see me again today. He writes here that you've been trying to lose weight and need some help in determining what factors have contributed to the lack of weight loss. Is that correct?" (The purpose of the initial response is to double-check the client's rationale for attending the interview.)

   CLIENT (fidgeting): "Well, that's true. Sometimes I think that all I have to do is to look at food and I gain weight."

Counselor thinks: She admits that she has a weight problem (indirectly). She seems to be discounting the contributing factors (distracting response). In frustration she tries to absolve herself from blame by attributing her problem to some unknown phenomenon that makes her gain weight at the very sight of food. For my next response I will check her thoughts as to her control over the weight gain.

2. COUNSELOR: "From what you have said you seem to think that your weight gain is out of your control. How well does that describe what you are thinking?"

   CLIENT: "Well, sometimes I feel that way but I suppose I do have some control."

Counselor thinks: Okay, the client is now admitting to having some control. I will focus next on areas where she may feel she has some control.

3. COUNSELOR: "What are some areas related to your weight gain that you do feel you can control?"

   CLIENT: "Well, I guess I could just stop buying groceries."

Counselor thinks: She either did not understand my question or she is feeling defensive about having to discuss situations where she might have control but doesn't exercise the option. My next response will focus on the idea of shopping and I will give her some examples using a self-disclosing response.

4. COUNSELOR: "Well, sometimes when I go shopping and I'm very hungry, I tend to buy more food and high-calorie snacks."

    CLIENT (voice pitch goes up, tone gets louder): "How would you know what it's like to go shopping and want foods you shouldn't have? You're not overweight."

Counselor thinks: My example seemed to make the client avoid the issue of contributing factors even more. She seems to have built up a great deal of frustration. Perhaps exploring her feelings about grocery buying might give me some clues. I will respond to her question and then direct the focus to her concern about buying groceries.

5. COUNSELOR: "I really can't know what it's like to be in your shoes. I can only express a situation similar to yours that I have been in. I guess buying groceries is a very important concern for you because it is tied so closely to your desire to lose weight. What feelings do you have while you're shopping?"

    CLIENT (loud voice): "I feel like a child in a candy store. Here is everything I love, everything that gives me pleasure, but I am forbidden to touch any of it. Then my kids and my husband are saying, 'Oh, go on honey (or mom) buy it; we love it. We shouldn't have to suffer just because you don't have any willpower.' "

Counselor thinks: That's the most I've gotten out of her. It's the first indication that she is willing to explore the situation. It seems that one of the factors contributing to her lack of ability to lose weight is her nonsupportive husband and children. I might check this theory out further.

6. COUNSELOR: "Are you saying that your family really doesn't give you a lot of support in losing weight?"

    CLIENT: "Yes. Being overweight is bad enough but when your own family gives you no support, losing weight is almost impossible."

Counselor thinks: The client seems to feel very strongly about this lack of family support. I will try to get at how this affects the way she feels in specific situations where nonsupport is apparent.

> 7. COUNSELOR: "Having your family respond negatively when you try to buy low-calorie foods and avoid high-calorie snacks seems to make you feel very frustrated. You would like them to praise your efforts. I guess having your family reject your efforts at weight loss may affect the way you see yourself, too."
>
> CLIENT (avoids eye contact): "What do you mean?"

Counselor thinks: From the lack of eye contact and the client's verbal message, I believe either my response was unclear or she isn't ready to look at her self-image yet. I will approach this indirectly by asking her to describe some situations in which she has felt frustrated by lack of support by her family.

> 8. COUNSELOR: "Well, I'm not sure. Maybe you could tell me exactly what happens in a situation where your family is nonsupportive."

At this point the interview enters the area where additional counseling skills are necessary. Chapter 3 discusses those skills and how they can help nutrition counselors in formulating plans and applying strategies during interviews.

NOTES

1. William H. Cormier and L. Sherilyn Cormier, *Interviewing Strategies for Helpers: A Guide to Assessment, Treatment and Evaluation* (Monterey, Calif.: Brooks/Cole Publishing Company, 1979), 11.

2. Ibid., 12–13.

3. Lawrence M. Brammer, *The Helping Relationship, Process and Skills* (Englewood Cliffs, N.J.: Prentice-Hall, 1979), 26–34.

4. John W. Loughary and Theresa M. Ripley, *Helping Others Help Themselves, A Guide to Counseling Skills* (New York: McGraw-Hill Book Company, 1979), 23–39.

5. Arthur Wright Combs et al., *Helping Relationships* (Boston: Allyn & Bacon, 1971), 10–17.

6. Leona E. Tyler, *The Work of the Counselor* (New York: Appleton-Century-Crofts, Educational Division, Meredith Corporation, 1969), 36–37.

7. Brammer, *Helping Relationship,* 36.

8. Robert R. Carkhuff and Richard M. Pierce, *The Art of Helping: Trainer's Guide* (Amherst, Mass.: Human Resources Development Press, 1975), 178–182.

9. Brammer, *Helping Relationship,* 24.

10. Cormier and Cormier, *Interviewing Strategies,* 31–40.

11. William R. Passons, *Gestalt Approaches in Counseling* (New York: Holt, Rinehart and Winston, 1975), 103–105.

12. Helen H. Gifft, Marjorie B. Washton, and Gail G. Harrison, *Nutrition, Behavior and Change* (Englewood Cliffs, N.J.: Prentice-Hall, 1972), 10–15.

13. Derald W. Sue and David Sue, "Barriers to Effective Cross-Cultural Counseling," *Journal of Counseling Psychology* 24 (1977): 427.

14. Cormier and Cormier, *Interviewing Strategies,* 43.

15. Ibid., 50.

16. Allen E. Ivey and Norma B. Gluckstern, *Basic Influencing Skills* (North Amherst, Mass.: Microcounseling Associates, 1976), 52–65.

17. John J. Lavelle, "Comparing the Effects of an Affective and a Behavioral Counselor Style on Client Interview Behavior," *Journal of Counseling Psychology* 24 (1977): 174.

18. Cormier and Cormier, *Interviewing Strategies,* 51.

19. Brammer, *Helping Relationship,* 81–83.

20. Cormier and Cormier, *Interviewing Strategies,* 77.

21. Ibid., 79.

22. Ibid.

23. Allen E. Ivey and Jerry Authier, *Microcounseling, Innovations in Interviewing, Counseling, Psychotherapy, and Psychoeducation* (Springfield, Ill.: Charles C Thomas, Publisher, 1978), 75.

24. Cormier and Cormier, *Interviewing Strategies,* 80.

25. Ibid., 81.

26. Ibid., 82.

27. Ibid., 84–85.

28. David W. Johnson, *Reaching Out: Interpersonal Effectiveness and Self-Actualization* (Englewood Cliffs, N.J.: Prentice-Hall, 1972), 159–172.

29. Ibid., 165.

30. Cormier and Cormier, *Interviewing Strategies,* 85.

31. Gerard Egan, *The Skilled Helper: A Model for Systematic Helping and Interpersonal Relating* (Monterey, Calif.: Brooks/Cole Publishing Company, 1975), 169–170.

32. Cormier and Cormier, *Interviewing Strategies,* 88.

33. Brammer, *Helping Relationship,* 94–95.

34. Ivey and Authier, *Microcounseling,* 113–115.

35. Cormier and Cormier, *Interviewing Strategies*, 95.

36. Vincenzo Giannandrea and Kevin C. Murphy, "Similarity in Self-Disclosure and Return for a Second Interview," *Journal of Counseling Psychology* 5 (1973): 547.

37. Brenda Mann and Kevin C. Murphy, "Timing of Self-Disclosure, Reciprocity of Self-Disclosure, and Reactions to an Initial Interview," *Journal of Counseling Psychology* 23 (1976): 306.

38. Norman R. Simonson, "The Impact of Therapist Disclosure on Patient Disclosure," *Journal of Counseling Psychology* 23 (1976): 5.

39. Ibid., 3.

40. Ibid.

41. Mary A. Hoffman-Graff, "Interviewer Use of Positive and Negative Self-Disclosure and Interviewer-Subject Sex Pairing," *Journal of Counseling Psychology* 24 (1977): 184.

42. Ibid., 185.

43. Ivey and Authier, *Microcounseling,* 111.

44. Cormier and Cormier, *Interviewing Strategies,* 101.

45. Arthur Schwartz and Israel Goldiamond, *Social Casework: A Behavioral Approach* (New York: Columbia University Press, 1975), 30.

46. Arnold P. Goldstein, "Relationship-Enhancement Methods," in *Helping People Change,* ed. Frederick H. Kanfer and Arnold P. Goldstein (New York: Pergamon Press, 1975), 19.

47. Arnold P. Goldstein, *Therapist-Patient Expectations in Psychotherapy* (New York: Pergamon Press, 1962), 121.

48. Cormier and Cormier, *Interviewing Strategies,* 107.

49. Ibid., 117.

50. Ibid., 118–124.

Chapter 3

Counseling Skills

Objectives for Chapter 3

1. Explain the counseling relationship.
2. Describe the counseling process.
3. Identify four types of data necessary for adequate nutrition assessment.
4. Describe the factors involved in nutrition need specification.
5. Apply six steps in goal definition in a given nutrition counseling problem.
6. List factors influencing diet adherence.
7. List predictors of poor adherence or nonadherence.
8. Apply at least two of five modeling strategies to help in solving a given nutrition problem.
9. Apply at least three of seven strategies designed to motivate behavior change for a given nutrition problem.
10. Apply at least two self-management strategies for a given nutrition problem.
11. Describe the purposes of evaluation.
12. List the steps in evaluation.
13. List three means of monitoring the client's nutrition behavior.
14. Describe the purpose in evaluating counselor performance.

3

INITIAL INFORMATION

A variety of skills form the loom upon which counseling abilities can be interwoven. Basic counseling skills can be categorized under these topics: initial information, assessment, treatment, and evaluation. The first step is providing initial information.

Structure

Stewart and his coworkers believe that explicit structure should be provided to all new clients.[1] The point at which that structure should be provided depends on the clients. Nutrition counselors should be aware of clients' feelings. If they seem anxious, unsure, hesitant, or insecure, practitioners should provide structure immediately. However, if they readily begin sharing a concern, providing structure at that time would be an intrusion on their thoughts so the counselors should introduce it later in the initial interview.

In describing the counseling process to clients, Stewart et al. recommend four aspects:

1. purpose
2. responsibility
3. focus
4. limits.[2]

Purpose

The purpose of counseling is to aid clients in coping with nutrition-related problems. The practitioners help them develop problem-solving skills to be used upon conclusion of the interview.

Responsibility

The counselors' responsibility to clients is to listen to their nutrition-related concerns and observe their behavior when discussing and reviewing diet records or histories. Counselors also interact with clients to provide a safe environment to try out new behavior.

Focus

The focus of the interviews is extremely important. Clients may present many concerns related to eating behavior but should be made aware that only one objective will be discussed at a time. However, before the interviews are finished, several objectives may be covered.

Limits

Nutrition counselors also should make clients aware that there are limits in counseling. Serious maladjustments should be reported to a psychologist or psychiatrist. Clients should know that the success of their counseling depends on their active participation. They also should be informed that all of the interviews will be confidential; any discussion of information with a third party would be undertaken only with their permission.

Most counseling programs require three or four visits, each of 30 to 60 minutes' duration. Interviews for evaluation and monitoring progress usually run 10 to 30 minutes. These are general guidelines. Each client is an individual, and the time required for counseling may vary depending on the problem.

ASSESSMENT

Collection of Data

As stated in Chapter 1, the assessment phase of counseling cannot be overemphasized. It should be the second step in the process. Mason and her coauthors describe four kinds of information collected in the assessment phase:

1. previous charting data
2. dietary intake data
3. environmental data
4. behavioral data[3]

Much of the biological information that can be collected will be found in previously charted data. Medical records can provide information on height and weight over time. Laboratory tests offer cues to general health status. Note should be made of specific laboratory determinations of nutrient levels and diagnosis or of specific reasons a client is seeking health care.

Extremely important to assessment is collection of dietary intake data, in which two important factors should be considered: (1) the types of nutrients consumed and (2) the appropriate quantities.[4]

Depending on the precision necessary, two methods can be used to assess the types of nutrients consumed. The *Daily Food Guide*, published by the U.S. Department of Agriculture, will give information on the food groups that are being consumed.[5] For more in-depth quantitative and qualitative information, diet histories are important. To analyze the data, food consumption tables can be used.

Determining the appropriateness of quantities consumed is not easy. Both the Recommended Dietary Allowances (RDA) and Canadian Dietary Standard (CDS) were developed originally to evaluate the dietary status of population groups. They were not intended to be used by nutrition counselors in evaluating individual dietary status.

Several factors should be considered in looking at quantities.[6] First is the variation among individuals. Second is the number of repetitive food intake assessments on individual clients. Third is the validity and reliability of the instruments used to collect data. An instrument is considered valid if it truly reflects the individual's nutritional status within the limitations set, i.e., time, place, etc. It is considered reliable if it consistently measures nutritional status, given the same limitations and criteria set initially. Many instruments developed for nutrition assessment have not been tested for either validity or reliability.

Environmental data can provide invaluable information for the assessment phase. Mason describes seven factors that may influence eating behaviors:

1. family status
2. occupation and income
3. education
4. ethnic orientation
5. religion
6. recreation
7. residence.[7]

Collection of eating behavioral data involves reviewing the stimulus for thought, the feeling connected with it, the resulting behavior, and its consequences. By reconstructing behavioral incidents in this way, it is possible to determine causes of behavior. It also may be of value to determine how behavior is maintained. Behavioral consequences may be positive or negative and may vary in intensity. Clients' reconstruction of these incidents can provide invaluable information for counselors. Ferguson offers a questionnaire that can provide insight into clients' eating behavior.[8] (See Appendix C)

Specification of Nutrition Needs

Client situations can be looked at in terms of specific problem behaviors.[9] After defining the difficulty in such terms, counselors should try to discover how the behaviors are influenced by the clients' environment. Behavior is affected by things happening within and outside oneself, by certain visible events (verbal, nonverbal, and motor responses), and by less visible events (thoughts, images, and physiological and affective states) that precede and follow many behaviors. These overt and covert happenings affect behavior by maintaining, increasing, decreasing, initiating, or eliminating it.

The ABC model of behavior identifies the relationship between the problem behavior and environmental events. In this model "B" is an example of behavior influenced by events that precede it (antecedent behavior, or "A") and events that follow (consequences, or "C").

Seven goals to work toward in defining a client's problems require counselors to:

1. explain the purpose of problem definition
2. identify and select the problem concerns
3. identify the present problem behaviors
4. identify the antecedent contributing conditions
5. identify the consequent contributing conditions
6. identify problem intensity
7. identify the coping skills.[10]

Selection of dietary problems to be confronted should involve mutual client and counselor agreement on the major concern. Related factors analyzed should include present problem behaviors, antecedent and consequent contributing conditions, problem intensity, and coping skills.

The counseling session ultimately must specify nutritional needs, cued by all of the factors just discussed. In the final analysis, clients obviously should be the central focus because they will be the primary change agents of both their behavior and their environment.

TREATMENT PLANNING

The third major step in counseling is formulating a treatment plan, which requires seven major steps.[11]

Goal Setting

A seven-step program for selecting goals is depicted in Figure 3–1. Nutrition counselors first should identify the purpose or goals of treatment, second, ask the clients to identify what change or result is desired from counseling, and, third, determine how realistic the positive aspects of the goal might be. Risks in achieving the goal might be delineated. An example of risk taking: an overweight husband reaches ideal weight but, because of the resulting improvement in appearance, his success produces resentment in his overweight wife who is worried about losing his affection to someone who likes him at the new, ideal weight.

The fourth step requires decision making. The clients may decide to reconsider making a change (weight loss may not be required), the counselors may decide to refer the individuals to a counseling psychologist, for example, or they may decide to work together toward achieving the goal. At this point clients and practitioners must define in specific terms the behavioral goal, the conditions and circumstances of change, the level or extent to which it should be achieved, and the degree to which the individuals will work to attain the goal. Subgoals also can be established.

Goals can have these attributes:

1. They are targets which indicate where to begin and where to finish.
2. They are motivators when explicitly stated and readily attainable.
3. They are rewarding.
4. They provide for planned change.[12]

The assumption that the problem or concern will provide a goal automatically is erroneous; it is up to clients and counselors together to identify the goal.

Goals provide direction and ambition but their achievement may be well beyond the ability of the clients and counselors. In the fifth step a behavior

Figure 3–1 Counselors' Steps in Selecting Dietary Goals with Client

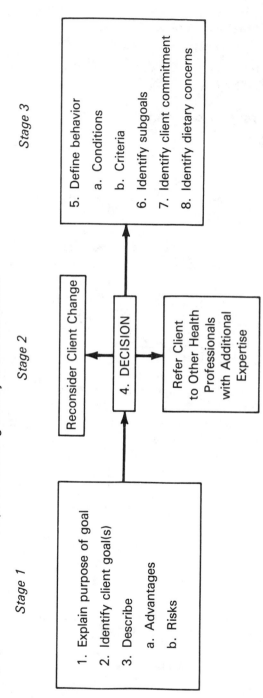

Stage 1   *Stage 2*   *Stage 3*

Source: Adapted from *Interviewing Strategies for Helpers* by William H. Cormier and L. Sherilyn Cormier, published by Brooks/Cole Publishing Company, Monterey, Calif., p. 166. Copyright © 1979 by permission of Brooks/Cole Publishing Company.

must be specified and incorporated into a subgoal to create focus and direction. Target behaviors should be specific, with conditions that put limits or constraints on performance of the conduct, along with minimum acceptable criteria or standards. Criteria might include a specific time during which the behavior should occur, a specific degree of performance, a description of task accomplishment, and the desired change of personal state.

The sixth step involves identification of specific subgoals. For example, setting a weight loss goal of 20 pounds in a year may be overwhelming to many clients. A subgoal of losing one pound every two weeks is more reasonable and gives them something to attain on a weekly basis. And finally, in the seventh step, client commitment is crucial to maintaining a dietary behavior.

Stewart et al. list three basic measures of client commitment:

1. The client has verbally agreed that the established goals are appropriate.
2. The counselor and client have discussed the costs of achieving the goal (e.g., time, money, risk, anxiety, embarrassment, etc.).
3. The client has verbalized commitment to work with this concern.[13]

Identifying Dietary Concerns

Once goal setting is complete, identifying dietary concerns (Figure 3–2) related to an objective and its subgoals is the next phase of the counseling process.

This stage of the process is crucial.[14] It is the joint responsibility of both parties to identify the dietary concerns the clients bring to the session—a process that will take considerable time. Dietary concerns may be related to spouse support, portion sizes, snacking, etc. To identify concerns the practitioners must maximize the use of both listening and probing skills.

From these many factors, clients and counselors must mutually identify the most immediate concern. Their selections can be based on a number of criteria such as the immediacy or complexity of the dietary problem. Often they may select the least complex concern first as it may be the easiest to achieve.

Nutrition counselors should focus on both the content and feelings expressed in the clients' verbalization. Stewart et al. point out that the content provides the counselor with information, actions, and objects. The feeling portion of verbalization can provide clues to attitudes concerning content.

Figure 3–2 Setting Up a Process for Dealing with Client Concerns

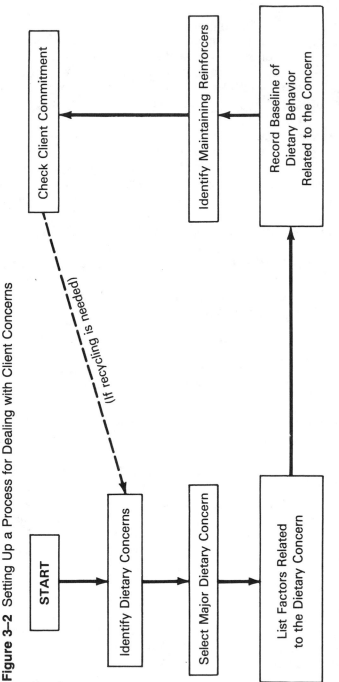

Source: Adapted from *Systematic Counseling* by Norman R. Stewart, Bob B. Winborn, Richard H. Johnson, Herbert M. Burks, Jr., James R. Engelkes, published by Prentice-Hall, Inc., p. 104. Copyright © 1978 by permission of Prentice-Hall, Inc.

It is important to differentiate between content and feeling because, by focusing separately on feelings with an affective response, counselors may move clients to further self-exploration.[15]

Analysis of responses to dietary questions demonstrates that they fall into four categories:

1. response component
2. temporal component
3. situational component
4. intensity component.[16]

This type of categorization can help in evaluating concerns in terms of the questions what, when, where, and how.

To identify the response facets of the problem, practitioners learn what the concern is, how it is demonstrated, and what effect it has on the client's life. It is the counselors' responsibility to describe the response in observable and measurable terms.

The temporal (timing) component of a dietary behavior can be immensely important. For this element, practitioners must be attuned to when the behavior occurs, how long it has occurred, and the sequence in which it emerges.

In the situational component the counselors try to determine where or under what circumstances the problem behavior occurs.

The fourth component, intensity, emphasizes the frequency or the number of times a dietary behavior occurs and its duration. Duration means the length of time over which a given dietary behavior occurs and how long it continues each time.

In many cases nutrition counselors spend too little time looking at baseline dietary behaviors. Baseline data provide an assessment of behavior in terms of situation, time, frequency, and duration. Client comments can provide some information but, ideally, a data gathering device is used to shed light on the current level of the dietary concern in terms of response, time, situation, and intensity. Two useful devices are a behavioral chart (Appendix D) and a behavioral log or record (Appendix E). Usually one to four weeks produce adequate baseline data. This type of reporting by clients can increase the accuracy of the data, strengthen their involvement, and give them encouragement because it provides for a feeling of self-control.[17]

Very important to eventual success is identification of which reinforcers promote dietary behaviors and which allow certain conduct to continue. Counselors will find it useful to list the benefits their clients derive from continuing certain behaviors that contribute to the dietary problem.[18] If clients can identify why a behavior persists, counseling can be more effective.

At this point, the counselors can double-check their accuracy in stating the dietary problem, its components, and the reinforcers that maintain or reduce it. Clients can amend, delete, or approve the process presented in Figure 3–2. Discrepancies between what counselors say and what clients think and feel can be discussed. A review of client interpretation of the dietary concern should cover the following:

1. concern definition
2. response component
3. temporal component
4. situational component
5. frequency component
6. maintaining component.[19]

Helping Strategies

Helping strategies are the plans of action designed to meet the specific goals of each client. Cormier and Cormier suggest these five guidelines for judging the timing for a helping strategy:

1. quality of the relationship
2. definition of the problem
3. development of desired counseling goals
4. client cues of readiness and commitment
5. collection of baseline measures.[20]

Mason et al. delineate a variety of factors necessary in selecting helping strategies. Focusing on goals is an obvious recommendation. Clients and counselors should use cues to stimulate appropriate responses and consequences that will reinforce desired behaviors. The strategy selected should help arrange more pleasant associations, with new thoughts and behaviors, and remove undesirable thoughts. The strategy should allow for trying the new behavior in an environment where it is likely to be reinforced positively.[21]

Factors Influencing Diet Adherence

In selecting helping strategies it is necessary to review factors that ultimately will influence client adherence to them. Four factors can be crucial to adherence: client, nutrition counselor, clinic, and regimen.[22]

The Role of the Client

The first factor involving the clients includes a variety of interview-related situations that are influential in adherence to a dietary pattern. Much of what takes place in a nutrition counseling session involves information giving to promote diet adherence. Research has shown that information recalled decreases in direct proportion to the amount given.[23] That study also shows that recall increases if information is presented over time rather than all at once. These researchers note that recall of information may be related to anxiety. Persons identified as having either high or low anxiety forget more than those with moderate anxiety; those with moderate anxiety show the best knowledge retention.

Studies also have looked at fear as a factor in retention of information.[24,25] The focus of these studies was the fear of complications of a disease. High levels of fear promote poor dietary adherence and may lead to inadequate nutrient intake descriptions.

In the author's experience, recall improves if information is categorized and each topic is presented to a client as a unit.

Research indicates that clients who live alone show poorer adherence to their diets.[26] In selecting helping strategies this factor should be weighed heavily.

Asymptomatic conditions requiring preventive or supportive treatment also tend to be associated with lower adherence rates.[27]

Persons who anticipate that a diet will be easy to follow may show poor adherence when those expectations are incongruent with their experience.[28] Experience has shown that when the family expects the client will adhere to the diet, performance is better.[29]

The Role of the Counselor

The client's satisfaction with care and with the nutrition counselor can influence adherence to diet. Several studies show an increase in adherence when satisfaction with both counselor and care is high.[30,31,32,33,34] It also has been shown that adherence increases if the client sees the same counselor at each visit.[35,36,37,38,39] It would seem that a personal nutrition counselor could individualize therapy more easily[40] and reduce feelings of anonymity.[41]

The Role of the Clinic

Clinic atmosphere also provides incentives for adherence to dietary strategies. A bright, well-lit room would seem to be more inviting than a dark, dingy one. A minimum of waiting time also would seem to be effective in helping to increase adherence.

The Role of the Regimen

The characteristics of dietary regimen also are crucial to maintaining good eating patterns. When many life changes are combined (diet, office habits, family, social functions, etc.), problems with adherence tend to increase.[42,43] The use of a life event inventory, including deaths in the family, retirement, divorce, etc., to assess life stresses may be helpful. Best adherence occurs when the initial dietary regimen is simple, with complexities introduced gradually. If problems arise, reassurance and inquiries about improvement can promote increased adherence. The following factors related to the regimen have been shown to affect adherence:

1. difficulty in fitting helping strategies into current life style
2. irregularity of the routine required by the helping strategies
3. difficulties with the regimen itself
4. carrying out the regimen at work or in a restaurant.[44]

The National Diet-Heart Study reported an inverse relationship between the frequency of restaurant eating and a fall in cholesterol.[45] In other words, whenever possible the regimen should be adapted to the client's life style.

Adherence Predictors

There are three possible predictors of adherence: attitudes, clinical judgment, and self-prediction. [46] Negative aspects associated with these factors, i.e., poor client attitudes, including predictions of low adherence, and nutritionists' preconceived negative judgments of the individuals, have been linked with future problems. However, they do not identify who will fail to follow any specific regimen; to date, no single factor has been pinpointed as an accurate adherence predictor.

Research shows that changes in beliefs are not related to alterations in long-standing diet patterns.[47] The performance of a given activity can predict subsequent adherence more clearly than can counselor attitudes or beliefs.

The second possible factor, the clinical judgment of the counselors as to whether or not adherence will be high or low, has not been shown to be effective in predicting compliance with a specific regimen.

Self-prediction of diet adherence has been reviewed by numerous researchers. In some cases clients are asked how well they could follow a regimen over time. Davis shows that while 77 percent of 154 new patients express a willingness to comply with their doctors' advice, only 63 percent actually exhibit compliant behavior.[48] Haynes et al. report that of subjects who agreed to participate in a blood pressure study, 38 of 230 did poorly in following a regimen and needed additional counseling in order to maintain adherence to blood pressure medication.[49] Davis, in a blood pressure study, finds that a simple interview will identify half of all nonadherers.[50] However, it must be emphasized that every client should be considered a potential nonadherer because the conditions that affect compliance will vary over time.

Several factors should be considered in deciding on a strategy, once a goal has been agreed upon. First, the counselors should study both objective and subjective data that may indicate client motivation and willingness to participate in carrying out the strategy, which must be one with which the practitioners feel comfortable.

Once the strategy has been selected, intermediate objectives to help in providing some degree of early success should be listed. These objectives should be reviewed carefully with the clients to be sure they are practical and attainable. Steps necessary to achieve them should then be delineated.

The next task is to list and perform the steps (sequenced learning). This does not mean that all of the burden of performance should fall on the clients. When reviewing what must be done to achieve the objectives, supporting or guiding activities by the counselors also should be listed. This part of sequenced learning is the single aspect that allows for behavior change; all other functions involve planning and assessing.

Steps for a Behavior Change Plan

Stewart et al., in listing six steps to promote learning and minimize failure, recommend that counselors:

1. divide nutrition information into manageable steps arranged in sequence
2. arrange for the first step in nutrition instruction to be managed with little effort
3. sequence the steps which follow so that the client is capable of attaining each one
4. attempt to make each step within the nutrition instruction small but not so easy or trivial that the client will consider it worthless
5. involve the client in planning changes in nutrition behaviors

6. state each step within the total nutrition instruction so that both client and counselor know what is expected and whether or not the step has been completed.[51]

In sequencing steps, counselors have a variety of alternatives in ordering each phase. There are essentially five types of sequences:

1. natural or logical sequence
2. sequences increasing in complexity
3. sequences increasing in frequency or duration
4. sequences decreasing in frequency or duration
5. sequences increasing in anxiety-producing stimuli.[52]

In counseling situations, client anxiety can play a large part in determining eventual change in eating behaviors. The client who is to begin a difficult goal behavior change may become so anxious over failure to meet the goal that progress stops. Instructional steps can be sequenced so that initial learning and practice occur in a nonthreatening interview such as in clients' role-playing situations with the counselors. Following this, situations holding progressively more potential threat in terms of behavioral change may be attempted.

For clients who are able to see the steps needed to reach their objectives, who can take the first one, and who are determined to follow the diet prescription over time, sequenced learning may be the only treatment strategy the nutrition counselors need to use. Stewart et al. provide a model of sequenced learning (Figure 3–3).[53] If the strategy steps have not been completed (step 6b on the flow chart), the process is repeated until success is achieved.

However, many clients cannot see clearly what is needed to solve their problem. Others may have fears that inhibit learning and following the diet. Still others may find it difficult to make a continued effort to follow through. In such situations, sequenced learning can be used but it is not enough—additional strategies must be selected, and the more that are available, the greater the likelihood of success.

Educational Focus for Improving Adherence

When the clients do not understand the purpose of the objectives or feel that they were set solely by the nutritionist, motivation decreases. Counselors also should pay particularly close attention to the difficulty and degree of challenge in each step.[54] In order to optimize behavior change, concrete actions to carry out the regimen, supervise practice, and indivi-

Figure 3–3 Model of Sequenced Learning

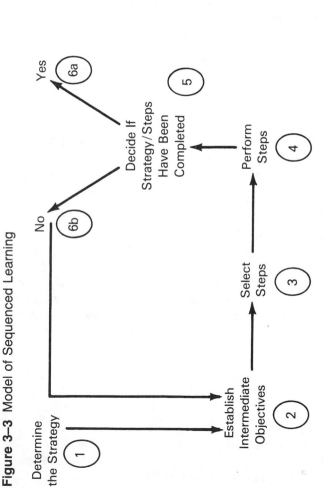

Source: Reprinted from *Systematic Counseling*, by Norman R. Stewart, Bob B. Winborn, Richard H. Johnson, Herbert M. Burks, Jr., and James R. Engelkes with permission of Prentice-Hall, © 1978, p. 135.

dualize instructions should be listed.[55] The major emphasis in an instructional plan should be to provide information about the regimen.

There are three facets to emphasize in instructing clients on an eating pattern: (1) information about the eating pattern itself, (2) how to construct the regimen around a day's activities, and (3) the rationale for its use. Providing information about the pattern itself may have limited value for future adherence[56] but careful instruction following the clients' suggestions as to how to fit the regimen into their daily activities should increase adherence over time[57,58,59] as well as provide the rationale for its use.[60] Behavior change in eating habits will be even more likely to occur if the counselors delineate a specific sequence of concrete actions,[61] allow for supervised practice of setting up a regimen,[62] and individualize the instruction for the unique circumstances of each client's life.[63,64]

STRATEGY IMPLEMENTATION

After a plan for treatment of a nutrition problem has been designed, a strategy or program for implementation—a vital part of counseling—must be set. A strategy is defined as a comprehensive plan for changing a client's existing eating behavior to a desired one. The majority of client and counselor time and effort will be devoted to this phase. To decrease time and produce more predictable results, a practical, uncomplicated strategy should be drawn up. Cormier and Cormier present a checklist for assuring the strategy is implemented (Exhibit 3–1).[65]

STRATEGIES FOR LEARNING NEW RESPONSES

Diet strategies obviously focus on a variety of problem situations. Some aim to help clients learn new responses, others may be designed to motivate behavior change, and still others seek to promote self-directed behavior.

Strategies to help promote new learning responses are modeling and simulation.

Modeling

Before presenting a model, the counselors must identify clearly the response to be learned and the situational variables in which it is to occur. Stewart et al. list several uses of modeling in counseling. Modeling is a procedure by which clients learn through observing and mimicking others. Modeling of a new response can increase client awareness of its perform-

Exhibit 3–1 Checklist for Implementing a Diet Strategy

A. Verbal Set for Strategy
  1. Did the nutrition counselor provide a rationale to the client about the strategy?
  2. Did the counselor give an overview of the strategy?
  3. Did the counselor obtain the client's willingness to try the strategy?
B. Modeling Goal Behavior
  1. Were instructions about what to look for in the modeled demonstration given to the client?
  2. Did the model demonstrate the goal behaviors in a coping manner?
  3. Was the modeled demonstration presented in a series of sequential scenarios?
  4. Did the client review or summarize the goal behaviors after the modeled demonstration?
C. Rehearsal of Goal Behaviors
  1. Did the counselor review target responses before practice attempts?
  2. Did the client engage in (a) covert rehearsal, (b) overt rehearsal, (c) both?
  3. In initial rehearsal attempts did the counselor provide coaching and/or induction aids (e.g., dietary maintenance tools)?
  4. Did the amount of coaching and induction aids decrease with practice attempts?
  5. Can self-directed practice of each goal behavior be observed?
  6. Was each practice attempt covered satisfactorily before moving on to another goal behavior? (Check which criteria were used in this decision):
    _____ the decision to move on was a joint one
    _____ client was able to enact the scene without feeling anxious
    _____ client was able to demonstrate target responses, as evidenced by demeanor and words
    _____ words and actions of the client were realistic to the onlooker
  7. Did the counselor and client go over or arrange for a taped playback of the rehearsal?
  8. Did the counselor give feedback to the client about the rehearsal? (Check whether counselor feedback included these elements):
    _____ positive reinforcer statement, a suggestion for improvement, and another positive reinforcer
    _____ the counselor encouraged each successive rehearsal attempt
D. Homework and Transfer of Training
  1. Assign rehearsal homework in the client's environment?
  2. Did the homework assignment include the following? (Check any that apply):
    _____ situations the client could easily initiate
    _____ graduated tasks: allow the client to gradually demonstrate the target response
    _____ a "do" statement for the client
    _____ a "quantity" statement for the client
  3. Was the client given self- or other-directed assistance in carrying out homework through:
    _____ written cue cards
    _____ a trained nutrition counselor aide
  4. Did the counselor instruct the client to make written self-recordings of both the strategy (homework) and the goal behaviors?
  5. Did the counselor arrange for a face-to-face or telephone follow-up after the client's completion of some of the homework?

Source: Adapted from *Interviewing Strategies for Helpers* by William H. Cormier and L. Sherilyn Cormier, published by Brooks/Cole Publishing Company, Monterey, Calif., pp. 275–276. Copyright © 1979, by permission of Brooks/Cole Publishing Company.

ance and behavioral outcome. Individuals need to incorporate new responses into a repertoire of those already learned.[66]

A second use of modeling is to demonstrate the practice of a behavior in a situation that in real life may be associated with fear, failure, anxiety, and pain.

There are several ways to set up modeling situations. The clients can be their own models. In such cases these individuals may model a behavior as it should occur, with the follow-up discussion focusing on why this sort of conduct cannot be actualized outside the counseling session. In other cases, the counselors can model a behavior if it is crucial for the clients to learn in order to solve a problem with eating behaviors. It may be helpful for the clinicians to point out environmental models, asking what persons in the clients' estimation have excellent eating behaviors. These then can be used as models.

Symbolic models may also be valuable. In this approach, the model is presented through written materials, audiotapes or videotapes, films, or slide-tape exercises. An example of a symbolic model might be an actor on videotape performing an appropriate response to a friend who was offering high-calorie foods on a special holiday such as at a Thanksgiving or religious feast.

Before a symbolic model is prepared, the practitioners should carefully consider the clients and their makeup. Of those who might be viewing, reading, or listening to the modeling, what are their average: age, sex, ethnic origin, cultural practices, coping, mastery of the model portrayed, and concerns or problems related to nutrition? Once the counselors have a good idea of the type of client who will be using the symbolic model, the goal behaviors to be modeled can be delineated. The medium could be a written script, audiotape, videotape, film, or slide-tape. The script should include instructions, modeled dialogue, practice, written feedback, written summarization of what has been modeled, and why it is important to the individual. Finally, the script should be field-tested on a sample of clients and modified on the basis of their comments and responses.[67]

Cormier and Cormier describe two additional types of modeling: covert[68] and emotive.[69] Covert modeling requires clients to use their imaginations. They are directed to imagine a model performing desired behaviors while being instructed. One advantage of this form is its low cost: no elaborate aids are necessary. It also permits a variety of problems to be addressed. The scenes of each modeling situation can be individualized to meet the concerns of specific clients. These same imaginary scenes also can be used to assist clients in practicing self-control in problem situations. With this form of modeling, clients can practice alone, an excellent alternative to live or filmed examples.

In the last form, emotive modeling, the clients focus on positive thoughts or images while imagining a discomfiting or anxiety-arousing activity or situation. By focusing on positive and pleasant images, they block embarrassing, fearful, or anxiety-provoking situations and learn possible ways to control responses and behavior in such settings.

Modeling seems best suited to nutritional problems that have characteristics such as these:

- The client is unaware of the response necessary to achieve an ultimate goal.
- The client is unfamiliar with the conditions that should cue a proper response.
- The client cannot foresee the reward potential of a proper response.
- The client may connect the response with a bad experience, making it unlikely that the performance will be attempted again.

Modeling provides a nonthreatening situation in which to perform a behavior. In threatening situations, individuals can establish avoidance reactions that inhibit learning a new response directly; the initial learning steps also can be nonrewarding or unpleasant. Modeling can allow the clients to learn the rewarding consequences of a behavior that they may have avoided previously.

Modeling is an excellent way to eliminate responses that may be inappropriate or used too frequently. During modeling an undesirable eating behavior can be identified and/or replaced by one that is more appropriate. Clients who present weak but relevant cues for certain behaviors can be shown how to intensify appropriate signals and reduce inappropriate or detrimental ones; they also can learn how to discern appropriate stimuli. Modeling is useful in helping clients acquire a single response or a complex pattern of behavior.

The script of modeling should reflect its content. Instructions should be given for each behavior to be demonstrated. The next part of the script should include a description of the behavior or activity to be modeled and possible dialogues of the model engaged in the activity. Following the modeling behaviors there should be opportunities for the clients to practice what they have just seen. Counselors should be prepared to give clients feedback on alternatives following practice. The script should also include a summary of what has been modeled and the importance of acquiring these behaviors.

Fidelity is essential in modeling: the effective model must be as close to the real situation as possible. This fidelity must be tempered with a provision for ease of management and control of stimuli in the counseling session.

Following the modeling situation, the counselors identify the relevant responses and situational cues for the clients. To make this follow-up more beneficial, preorganizers or an outline to identify important elements being modeled should be provided. During the modeling, stopping the client during the action for commentary can help in explaining a response. It is sometimes helpful to prepare a script with clients so that careful thought can go into their responses. In preparing a modeling script (see Exhibit 3–2) it may be of value to exaggerate important aspects and reduce extraneous elements.

Before the modeling, a typed sheet of preorganizers can be handed to the client and discussed. While watching the modeling, the client might be asked to keep the following preorganizer questions in mind:

- What precipitated the model's response?
- What were the situational conditions and social stimuli?
- What was said?
- What was the manner of speech?
- What did the model do?
- What were the consequences of the model's response?
- How did others react?
- How did the model seem to feel about the experience?

Exhibit 3–2 Modeling Script

- *Instructions:* Target behavior is to eat wisely at parties.
- *Description of the Behavior:* The model is attending a graduation party where both high- and low-calorie foods are served and should use an appropriate response to an offer of high-fat foods.
- *Possible Dialogues:*
    Host: "Hey, Joe, have some of these cheese chips! They're great!"
    Guest: "No, thanks, Bob. I'm trying to avoid high-fat snacks. These fresh vegetables look perfect! Think I'll try some."
- *Discussion of Practice Alternatives*
- *Summary:* This modeled situation offered an example of how one might respond at a party to offers of inappropriate foods. Alternatives have been discussed. The actual use of this modeled behavior can assist the client in routinely following a dietary pattern, even during parties.

More specific questions could be added for each individual nutrition counseling case.

SIMULATION

Simulation is a convenient strategy for providing opportunities for clients to try out responses. In modeling, clients observe and learn behaviors; in simulation, they act as participants. Simulation provides a safe environment for experiencing new responses. It is preferred to an actual situation for several reasons:[70]

- It allows individuals (clients or counselors) to cause events to happen.
- It makes it possible to compress time.
- It provides conditions that can be simplified to focus on one or two variables at a time.
- It enables conditions to be controlled so that learning is managed more easily than in real-life encounters.

Stewart et al. delineate three types of simulation: (1) role playing; (2) decision-making practice, in which groups can be formed, with each member identifying with the case so individual clients then can see how the others would handle a problem; (3) learning games.[71]

Simulations have a variety of uses in counseling. They can help in diagnosing existing or potential problems. In many cases, with clients who have no idea what is contributing to their inappropriate eating behaviors, simulation can reveal relevant aspects of the problems and stimulate the persons to recall vital elements. This strategy also permits trying alternate responses and evaluating the acquisition of new replies.[72]

Stewart et al. list seven techniques necessary to develop and use this strategy. They advise counselors to:

1. Begin by listing responses and environmental elements necessary in the simulation.
2. Carefully work as a client-counselor team to develop the situation and roles.
3. Discuss with the client the roles, situational elements, and the purposes of the simulation.
4. Act out the simulation.

5. Debrief the client. Ask the client to recall experiences and observations. Discuss relevant aspects of the client's performance.
6. Reenact the simulation with [the] modifications discussed following the first trial. Vary the simulation to promote the generalization of learning.

Continue the process until the objective of the simulation has been reached.[73]

MOTIVATING BEHAVIOR CHANGE

There are a number of strategies for motivating behavior change: thought stopping, cognitive restructuring, reinforcement, extinction, tailoring, shaping, and contracting.

Thought Stopping

Thought stopping is useful in controlling unproductive or self-defeating thoughts and images by suppressing or eliminating these negative cognitions. Although thought stopping has been used widely and clinical case studies show encouraging results, there is little empirical evidence available from controlled investigations to support the procedure. The advantages of this procedure are that it is easily administered and that clients usually understand and use it readily in a self-regulatory manner.[74]

A two-step sequence is presented for thought stopping:

1. The client allows any thoughts related to eating behavior to come to mind.
2. When the client notices a self-defeating thought, the client stops by covertly saying, "Stop!"[75]

This process is repeated until the client is able to avert self-defeating thoughts with only the covert interruption.

Rimm and Masters suggest that clients think positive thoughts after the self-defeating ones are interrupted; essentially, they learn to replace negative thoughts with positive, self-directed ones following the interruption.[76] In lieu of using assertive thoughts, the clients can be asked to focus on a pleasurable or reinforcing scene[77,78,79] or a neutral scene, such as an object in the environment.[80]

Mahoney and Mahoney suggest stopping a chain of self-defeating thoughts by replacing them with self-reinforcing ones.[81] For example, a negative monologue might go like this:

"If it weren't for my job and my family, I could lose weight."

An appropriate monologue to substitute might be:

"My schedule isn't any more hectic than anyone else's. I will be more creative in the ways I try to improve my eating habits."

Nutrition counselors can request that the clients practice this behavior at home using log sheets (Appendix F) to record the number of times they used thought stopping[82] and the kinds of negative thoughts and positive ones that were used as replacements.[83] During the subsequent interview the log sheets should be reviewed carefully. Positive reinforcement for completing the log regardless of its content is important, particularly for positive thoughts used to replace negative ones. The counselor should work with the client in deciding on how to change negative monologues.

Cognitive Restructuring

Another very similar strategy is cognitive restructuring. This involves using coping thoughts to replace negative or self-defeating ones. There is a great deal of similarity between the assertive thoughts described by Rimm and Masters[84] and the types of thoughts proposed in cognitive restructuring.

Cormier and Cormier describe six steps necessary in the use of cognitive restructuring during a client interview. The counselors should:

1. provide a rationale and overview of the procedure
2. identify client thoughts during problem situations
3. introduce and practice coping thoughts
4. shift from self-defeating to coping thoughts
5. introduce and practice positive or reinforcing self-statements
6. complete homework and do follow-up.[85]

Examples of self-defeating and coping thoughts are provided in Chapters 4 through 9. Appendix G is an example of a daily record for listing use of cognitive restructuring.

Reinforcement

Reinforcement is a crucial strategy for motivating change in eating behaviors. The likelihood of an appropriate eating behavior recurring depends upon the consequences. Reinforced desirable behaviors will be more likely to recur than unreinforced ones.

B.F. Skinner is credited with providing most of the basic research on the influence of reinforcement on learning.[86] A desired response can be taught through a process called shaping (discussed later in this chapter). In shaping, successive approximations of the desired response are rewarded until the new behavior is learned. Consequences of a response can increase or decrease the likelihood of its recurring.[87,88]

The management of reinforcement has been referred to as behavior modification. Research has shown that behavior modification is useful in eliminating inappropriate behaviors and in producing goal-directed responses.[89,90,91]

Reinforcement can be used effectively in counseling by identifying the response to be reinforced, selecting the appropriate reinforcers, and having someone monitor and dispense them at the proper time.

Counselors begin by identifying the responses that will be reinforced, then clearly describe both the behavior and the circumstances under which they are to be performed. A quantity also should be affixed to the reinforcement. It also is necessary to decide which will be reinforced—each occurrence of the behavior or the persistence with which clients perform a response for a period of time.

A system should be set up whereby appropriate eating behaviors are reinforced immediately; however, if this is impossible, rewarding the end product of a series of such behaviors can be effective.

Reinforcement can take many forms. Social reinforcement can involve approval through verbal or nonverbal signs by a person, group, spouse, family, and/or peers.

Giving clients information on past performance can be reinforcing. Arranging information on future performance in small steps that the learners can accomplish is important in helping to increase positive reinforcement.[92]

In some instances it is possible to use tangible reinforcement such as money, clothes, etc., or valueless tokens that can be exchanged for some object or privilege related to eating behavior.

Physical activities such as swimming, hiking, and skiing are extremely important reinforcers. They not only act as reward systems but also help increase caloric expenditure, firm muscles, and decrease appetite (if the exercise is strenuous).

Reinforcement also can be covert or imaginal, which helps clients remain self-directed. This also is discussed later in the chapter.

All of these types of reinforcers are affected by deprivation or satiation. If there has been a period of deprivation of a reinforcer before its administration, its influence will be increased.[93] Rewards that are readily available are poor motivators.

The agents providing reinforcement can vary. Counselors, clients, or significant others in their environment all should be considered possible reinforcing agents.

Nutrition counselors should make several judgments before deciding when to reinforce clients. While they are learning new eating behaviors, frequent rewards are most effective.[94] Each occurrence of a new behavior or each step toward it should be reinforced. During the initial learning period, rewards should be dispensed often and regularly in order to help the clients learn to associate the appropriate eating behavior with the compensation.

As progress is made, reinforcement should be administered less frequently and on a variable schedule, leading ultimately to fading. A varying number of unrewarded responses can be allowed to occur between those that are rewarded. As noted earlier, it is best to dispense the reward immediately following appropriate behavior.

Reinforcement is indicated in nutrition counseling when the following conditions exist:

- when the eating behavior to be learned requires a great deal of practice before it can become a habit
- when the initial learning attempts are painful
- when the actual rewards that come with a new eating behavior are far off.

By using reinforcement selectively, the counselors place some of the responsibility for the situation and the solution in the clients' hands.

Extinction

How can nutrition counselors stop unwanted eating behaviors? A strategy called extinction offers some clues.

An unwanted behavior persists because it is reinforced. In the same way, that eating pattern gains attention, reduces anxiety, or rewards the individual. To eliminate the behavior, the counselors must eliminate the reward. When withdrawal or prevention of reinforcement occurs, extinction of the behavior follows. Clients can be asked to avoid certain group situations where inappropriate eating behaviors are reinforced. Another extinction method is called satiation, in which the conduct is repeated again and again, well beyond the point of fatigue. However, this is recommended only as a last resort.

The extinction strategy begins with identification of the maintaining reinforcement. When and under what circumstances the eating behavior occurs, including conditions that make it more intense or more frequent, and its immediate consequences, are recorded. Factors that appear to reduce the behavior should be noted. The clients are asked the following questions:

1. When you are eating inappropriately, what happens?
2. How do others react?
3. How do you feel?

Unwanted eating behaviors must be extinguished in the settings in which they normally occur. Implementation of extinction can be very time consuming, in part because the clients' immediate reaction may even be to increase the behavior.

Tailoring

Tailoring, another strategy designed to motivate change, refers to the process of fitting the behavior to the clients' daily routine. This minimizes the number of changes the individuals must make. When using this strategy, close attention is paid to the initial baseline diet history. It often is possible to meet a dietary prescription and still arrange the eating pattern in accord with the clients' life styles and past patterns.

There are several very valid assumptions behind this strategy. First, it presumes that health behaviors are carried out in a total life context and therefore are affected directly by various aspects of daily living. It also assumes that there is no standard dietary pattern for a standard client but that each individual has unique circumstances to which the therapy must be adapted.[95]

Shaping

Shaping is a strategy that involves a gradual building of skills necessary to change a behavior. The clients proceed in steps to achieve the set criterion and gradually reach full performance. For example, cholesterol intake would be reduced from 300 milligrams a day to 200 milligrams, then 100 milligrams.

The graduated approach[96] is very similar to the shaping strategy. In the graduated approach, steps proceed from simple to complex behaviors and build upon one another. Important to this approach is starting at the clients' existing levels of performance. (Implementation of this approach is discussed in Chapters 4 through 9.)

Contracting

The last strategy for motivating behavior change, contracting, involves a written agreement between the nutrition counselors and the clients. The agreement is signed by both parties and includes the clients' agreement to carry out certain behaviors with rewards and/or punishment contingent on performance. As noted, money or other valuables sometimes are used as reinforcers. With this strategy, clients play a large role in designing their own treatment. Counselors provide advice and support while encouraging the clients to plan and implement a self-managed treatment.

There are several advantages to using the contracting strategy.[97,98,99] Because the contract is in writing, this provides a hard-copy outline of expected behaviors.[100] Client control over treatment permits discussion of potential solutions as well as problems. The contract constitutes formal commitment to the treatment. It also provides incentive value through the establishment of rewards from self or others for attaining goals.

STRATEGIES FOR BECOMING SELF-DIRECTED

Eventually what all nutrition counselors strive for is clients who are self-directed. The next two strategies, decision making and self-management, help in promoting self-direction.

Nutrition counseling is merely a brief encounter in clients' lives and its effects can be severely limited unless the individuals achieve increased control over their behavior. When clients become more self-directed, the practitioners are approaching a form of preventive counseling by preparing these persons for coping with anticipated problems on their own.

Decision Making

Clients and counselors work through the following sequence to help in making decisions to facilitate change in eating behaviors that have been causing problems. First, the problem is identified by the clients' answers to the following questions.

1. What is the inappropriate eating behavior?
2. What interferes with a solution?
3. When does the eating behavior occur?
4. In what situations does the eating behavior occur?
5. Under what circumstances does the eating behavior occur?
6. Under what conditions is the eating behavior most or least in variance from the recommended dietary pattern?

> 7. When must a decision be made or the problem eating be-
>   havior resolved?
> 8. How much effort is necessary to find a solution?
> 9. What behaviors contribute to the problem or interfere with
>   its solution?
> 10. What evidence will indicate that the inappropriate eating
>   behavior has been extinguished?[101]

Once these are answered, both values and goals must be reevaluated. Not all solutions will be acceptable to clients. Their values and goals as they relate to the problem are examined so that the solution sought will be compatible with those factors. The clients might then generate a list of possible solutions or alternative courses of action. Each alternative should be evaluated in terms of time, money, effort, and advantages and disadvantages. The clients begin moving toward a solution by tentatively choosing some course of action. (It may be necessary to reexamine the decision later and select a new course.)

There are several indicators that can help nutrition counselors in determining whether or not to use decision making as a strategy.[102] First, decision making will be of value if the clients are concerned about a choice to be made or an eating problem to be resolved and are unaware of alternatives. It also may be of benefit for those who lack the information to decide among alternatives or who lack a method for systematically examining options and making decisions.

Decision making really is an information-processing operation.[103] The nutrition counselors' task is to help clients achieve accurate self-information and feedback. By looking at past personal experience involving specific eating behaviors, the clients can discover values, interests, and abilities.

SELF-MANAGEMENT

Strategies for self-management involve self-monitoring, stimulus control, alternate responses, and altering the consequences of replies. It requires clients to alter their eating patterns on their own.

Self-Monitoring

Through self-monitoring using a food diary and intake graphs or charts, clients can learn more about their specific existing eating behaviors. Role playing also can be a valuable way of reviewing eating patterns. Counselors and clients can role play, record it, and discuss it immediately, using the tape recording as an instant replay.

Self-information can come from those around the clients. Nutrition counselors may need to confront them at times with information about eating habits that they may not have noticed.

Client decision making and use of self-information are excellent motivators because they help these individuals see themselves as having control over their behavior. Clients can monitor their progress even while alone; in some cases, only they can analyze thoughts about eating behavior. The decision-making strategy can be applied to future eating problems and can help prevent inappropriate behaviors before they arise.[104]

Self-management is crucial to the process of becoming self-directed. Counselors begin by collecting baseline information from clients' self-observation, recording relevant eating behaviors, the circumstances under which they occur, their frequency, duration, and other pertinent aspects. Clients should record this baseline information as soon as it occurs, not from memory.[105]

Clients also should note the location, time during the day, and the conditions in which the responses occur most frequently. In weight-control programs, self-monitoring may need to become a life-long commitment.

Stimulus Control

Clients also must control the environmental stimuli associated with an eating behavior in order to be self-directed. All of their dietary behaviors are influenced by such stimuli. Situational factors can become cues that evoke or control particular behaviors. By no means can all problems be solved by avoiding situations or finding new environments.

Nutrition counselors must make clients aware that there are two types of eating patterns that may cause problems.[106] First is the habitual behavior that is inappropriate and in need of modification. In such cases a way must be found to interrupt the normal chain of events. Cueing is one way of accomplishing this. Cues should be attention getting and should be associated as closely as possible with normal environmental stimuli that can evoke the response later when the special cue no longer is used. Self-cueing involves associating a response with environmental cues to effect long-term change in eating behaviors. For the client following a cholesterol-modified eating pattern, notes on the refrigerator emphasizing the use of vegetables as snack foods may serve as cues. Another example of a cue would be a written reminder on the calendar emphasizing daily exercise for the client trying to lose weight.

A second type of eating behavior requires stimulus control for modification of conduct that is excessive or inappropriate. To control this type of conduct, the environmental stimuli under which it is permitted to occur may be reduced gradually until it is performed only in an appropriate time and place.

By gradually increasing the time spent on an appropriate eating behavior in the selected environment, the stimulus value of the setting is strengthened. The setting helps elicit the desired response. The effort is to disassociate an eating behavior from a particular stimulus. This is accomplished by gradually eliminating the setting in which the response to be controlled tends to occur or by selecting one in which all responses but the controlled one are disallowed.

Interrupting response chains also can alter stimuli that elicit unwanted eating behaviors. If the chain is disrupted in its early stage, the series of inappropriate behaviors cannot lead automatically to the terminal unwanted response.

Stewart et al. recommend counselors take these three steps in controlling stimuli:

1. identify elements in the eating behavior chain
2. alter conditions at one or preferably many points
3. interrupt the chain early in the sequence.[107]

Alternate Responses

In self-management the clients must identify the situation in which the undesired eating behavior occurs and develop alternate patterns in each. Cueing may be necessary to remind them to use the alternate behaviors until the new conduct becomes associated with the natural environmental cues.

Altering Response Consequences

Individuals using self-rewards must learn to modify their eating behavior by monitoring their own responses and to reward reactions they see as being goal directed.

When self-direction is being implemented, Stewart et al. recommend strategies using covert responses (thoughts, feelings, imagery, and attitudes).[108] They suggest using thoughts as target behaviors. Clients begin by identifying desirable self-statements, monitor the frequency of positive self-thoughts, use a cue to elicit the desired ones, and finally reinforce the positive ones.[109]

In covert modeling, clients anticipate a difficult interaction and develop an imagined model of the response desired. They then rehearse covertly by imagining performing the model response in a variety of appropriate settings. When small successes are achieved, they think positive self-thoughts. This process is called covert reinforcement. A further step can be labeled covert sensitization. In that process, clients link undesirable eating behaviors with an imagined aversive consequence. This is thought to be effective in reducing the actual incidence of an inappropriate response.[110]

EVALUATION

Evaluation of clients' progress by client and counselor and counselor self-evaluation provides a very important conclusion to a nutrition counseling session. It has two purposes: (1) to determine clients' progress, and (2) to improve counselors' effectiveness in dealing with future clients or in further activities with present ones.[111]

Nature of Evaluation

The focus of nutrition counseling should be the clients' behavior—what they actually do as a result of the processs—not their feelings, attitudes, or self-concept except as those factors are affected by modifications in the individuals' eating behavior.

A review of client performance includes analyzing outcomes, determining whether or not the objectives were reached, and deciding on the need for additional counseling.[112] Some questions counselors might ask themselves are:

1. Did the client achieve the objectives as efficiently and completely as possible?
2. What have I learned from the nutrition counseling session to use in future situations?[113]

Steps in Evaluation

Evaluation is a continuous processing of behavioral information. Counselors should begin by evaluating the accomplishment of intermediate objectives, then what the clients have done following the sessions. Evaluation strategies should be based on the clients' reports, outside sources if necessary, and clues from role-play situations.[114]

Clients should be asked to provide a record of their eating behaviors that should be compared with the objectives.[115] If the objectives were attained, counselors should decide whether further sessions are necessary by determining whether the clients are motivated enough to continue current appropriate eating behaviors on their own. Another concern or a new aspect of the same concern should be identified and the desired objective related to it. In some cases if the objective was reached there may be no need to go on.[116]

Monitoring Client Performance

Three methods of measuring clients' degree of adherence to a diet program are:

1. client interviews
2. biochemical analysis.
3. daily records.[117]

The outcome of treatment should not be used as an indicator of how well clients are adhering to their diets. For example, weight loss should not be used as the only indication that they are following a low-calorie diet. Rather, the behavior necessary to decrease food intake can be used as one indicator of adherence. No one completely reliable measure of adherence has yet been identified so information must be obtained from a variety of sources.

The validity of client interviews depends upon the skill of the counselors and how well they can assess behavior. Validity also depends on the clients' memory and willingness to report dietary adherence behaviors honestly. Research indicates that nonadherence is underreported.[118] Reliability tends to improve if the patients are aware that their behavior is being assessed.[119] Overestimation of dietary intake often occurs with low consumption, underestimation is more frequent with high consumption. Specific features of the diet—calories, protein, and vitamins—also may be misreported.[120]

Biochemical assessment (through analysis of metabolic products of a dietary alteration or of the therapeutic substance itself in serum or urine) provides a more direct means of measuring adherence but does not tend to be adequate over time.[121] Biochemical methods at best provide little information on the current degree of adherence, and individual variations may give misleading values.[122] The National Diet-Heart Study reports a low correlation between biochemical measures and nutritionists' ratings (.05 to .47). Such wide individual variations decrease the reliability and usefulness of biochemical assessment.[123]

Daily records, as a means of assessing treatment progress, have been used in behavioral weight-control programs.[124] The clients record the amount and kind of foods consumed along with the time of eating and related circumstances. The literature reports several time periods for dietary recording:

1. an initial and final seven-day food record
2. two two-week food records
3. a weighed food record one day a week for seven weeks and one day a month thereafter for five years.[125,126,127]

In evaluating records, counselors must keep in mind the possibility of errors in estimating portion size or omission of items.[128] The advantage of dietary records includes the continuous generation of data on the behaviors under investigation. Records can provide information on erratic performance and on the origin of problems within a dietary regimen.[129] Some nutritionists find it useful to request clients to keep food records as they maintain the diet. The process of writing down foods eaten forces the clients to focus on what they are consuming and stimulates dietary adherence.

Evaluating Counselor Performance

The last step in the evaluation process pertains to counselor performance. Questions a counselor might ask include:

1. Did I help the client achieve the original objective as quickly as possible?
2. Did I use the most effective strategy?
3. Could my client have been more efficiently served by a referral source [i.e., a counseling psychologist]?
4. Were my counseling techniques appropriate for this particular client?[130]

NOTES

1. Norman R. Stewart et al., *Systematic Counseling* (Englewood Cliffs, N.J.: Prentice-Hall, 1978), 95–97.

2. Ibid., 97–103.

3. Marion Mason, Burness G. Wenberg, and P. Kay Welsch, *The Dynamics of Clinical Dietetics* (New York: John Wiley & Sons, 1977), 143–144.

4. Ibid., 144.

5. *Daily Food Guide* (Washington, D.C.: U.S. Department of Agriculture, Agricultural Research Service, Food and Nutrition Service, FNS–13, July 1975).

6. Mason et al., *Dynamics,* 154–155.

7. Ibid., 156–158.

8. James M. Ferguson, *Learning to Eat, Behavior Modification for Weight Control—Leader Manual* (Palo Alto, Calif.: Bull Publishing Company, 1975), Appendix—Eating Questionnaire.

9. William H. Cormier and L. Sherilyn Cormier, *Interviewing Strategies for Helpers: A Guide to Assessment, Treatment, and Evaluation* (Monterey, Calif.: Brooks/Cole Publishing Company, 1979), 128–131.

10. Ibid., 140.

11. Ibid., 165–166.

12. Stewart et al., *Systematic Counseling,* 115–132.

13. Ibid., 131.

14. Ibid., 103.

15. Ibid., 103–106.

16. Ibid., 106–108.

17. Ibid., 109–110.

18. Ibid., 110–111.

19. Ibid., 111–113.

20. Cormier and Cormier, *Interviewing Strategies,* 251–252.

21. Mason, Wenberg, and Welsch, *Dynamics,* 207–209.

22. Foods and Nutrition Resource Center, ed., *Nutrition Counseling Manual for Lipid Research Clinic Nutritionists* (Iowa City, Iowa: University of Iowa Printing Service, 1980), 43.

23. C.R.B. Joyce et al., "Quantitative Study of Doctor-Patient Communication," *Quarterly Journal of Medicine* 38 (1969): 183–194.

24. L. Holder, "Effects of Source, Message, Audience Characteristics on Health Behavior Compliance," *Health Service Representative* 87 (1972): 843–850.

25. Howard Leventhal, "Changing Attitudes and Habits to Reduce Risk Factors in Chronic Disease," *American Journal of Cardiology* 31 (1973): 571–580.

26. Morton Archer, Seymour Ringles, and George Christakis, "Social Factors Affecting Participation in a Study of Diet and Coronary Heart Disease," *Journal of Health and Social Behavior* 8 (1967): 22–31.

27. Barry Blackwell, "Drug Therapy: Patient Compliance," *New England Journal of Medicine* 289 (1973): 249–252.

28. Jacqueline M. Dunbar, "Adherence to Medication Regimen: An Intervention Study with Poor Adherers" (Ph.D. diss., Stanford University, 1977), 13.

29. Ibid., 19.

30. Richard L. Hagen, John P. Foreyt, and Thomas W. Durham, "The Dropout Problem: Reducing Attrition In Obesity Research," *Behavior Therapy* 7 (1976): 463–471.

31. Barbara S. Hulka et al., "Satisfaction with Medical Care in a Low Income Population," *Journal of Chronic Disease* 24 (1971): 661–673.

32. Arnold V. Hurtado, Merwyn R. Greenlick, and Theodore J. Colombo, "Determinants of Medical Care Utilization: Failure to Keep Appointments," *Medical Care* 11 (1973): 189–198.

33. P.R. Kaim-Caudle and G.N. Marsh, "Patient-Satisfaction Survey in General Practice," *British Medical Journal* 1 (1975): 262–264.

34. J.A. Kincey et al., "Patient Satisfaction in General Practice," *British Medical Journal* 3 (1975): 97–98.

35. J.J. Alpert, "Broken Appointments," *Pediatrics* 53 (1964): 127–132.

36. David L. Sackett and R. Brian Haynes, ed., *Compliance with Therapeutic Regimens* (Baltimore: The Johns Hopkins University Press, 1976), 40–50.

37. Marshall H. Becker, Robert H. Drachman, and John R. Kirscht, "Predicting Mother's Compliance with Pediatric Medical Regimens," *Journal of Pediatrics* 81 (1972): 843–845.

38. Marshall H. Becker and Lois A. Maiman, "Sociobehavioral Determinants of Compliance with Health and Medical Care Recommendations," *Medical Care* 13 (1975): 10–24.

39. John R. Caldwell et al., "The Dropout Problem in Antihypertensive Treatment," *Journal of Chronic Disease* 22 (1970): 579–592.

40. Evan Charney, "Patient-Doctor Communication: Implications for the Clinician," *Pediatric Clinics of North America* 19 (1972): 263–279.

41. John F. Rockart and Paul B. Hofmann, "Physician and Patient Behavior Under Different Scheduling Systems in a Hospital Outpatient Department," *Medical Care* 7 (1969): 463–470.

42. M.S. Davis and R.L. Eichhorn, "Compliance with Medical Regimens: A Panel Study," *Journal of Health and Social Behavior* 4 (1963): 240–249.

43. Walter J. Johannsen, George A. Hellmuth, and Thomas Sorauf, "On Accepting Medical Recommendations: Experiences with Patients in a Cardiac Work Classification Unit," *Archives of Environmental Health* 12 (1966): 63–69.

44. Dunbar, *Medication Regimen,* 19–22.

45. National Diet-Heart Study, "Final Report," *Circulation,* March 1968, Supplement no. 1.

46. Foods and Nutrition Resource Center, *Counseling Manual,* 51.

47. Ibid.

48. Milton S. Davis, "Physiologic, Psychological and Demographic Factors in Patient Compliance with Doctor's Orders," *Medical Care* 6 (1968): 115–122.

49. R. Brian Haynes et al., "Improvement of Medication Compliance in Uncontrolled Hypertension," *Lancet* 1 (1976): 1265–1268.

50. Davis, "Physiologic Factors."

51. Stewart et al., *Systematic Counseling,* 136.

52. Ibid., 137–138.

53. Ibid., 135.

54. Ibid., 144.

55. Foods and Nutrition Resource Center, *Counseling Manual,* 64, 66.

56. David L. Sackett et al., "Randomized Clinical Trial of Strategies for Improving Medication on Compliance in Primary Hypertension," *Lancet* 1 (1975): 1205–1207.

57. F.F. Dickey, M.E. Mattar, and G.M. Chudzek, "Pharmacist Counseling Increases Drug Regimen Compliance," *Hospitals* 49 (1975): 85–88.

58. Joseph A. Linkewich, Robert B. Catalano, and Herbert L. Flack, "The Effect of Packaging and Instruction on Outpatient Compliance with Medication Regimens," *Drug Intelligence and Clinical Pharmacy* 8 (1974): 10–15.

59. James M. McKenney et al., "The Effect of Clinical Pharmacy Services on Patients with Essential Hypertension," *Circulation* 48 (1973): 1104–1111.

60. Irving S. Colcher and James W. Bass, "Penicillin Treatment of Streptococcal Pharyngitis: A Comparison of Schedules and the Role of Specific Counseling," *Journal of the American Medical Association* 222 (1972): 657–659.

61. Leventhal, "Changing Attitudes."

62. Rhoda G. Bowen, Rosemary Rich, and Rozella M. Schlotfeldt, "Effects of Organized Instruction for Patients with the Diagnosis of Diabetes Mellitus," *Nursing Research* 10 (1961): 151–159.

63. Jeanne C. Hallburg, "Teaching Patients Self-Care," *Nursing Clinics of North America* 5 (1970): 223–231.

64. S.G. Rosenberg, "Patient Education Leads to Better Care for Heart Patients," *HSMHA Health Reports* 86 (1971): 793–802.

65. Cormier and Cormier, *Interviewing Strategies*, 275–276.

66. Stewart et al., *Systematic Counseling*, 148–161.

67. Cormier and Cormier, *Interviewing Strategies*, 278–280, 296.

68. Ibid., 307.

69. Ibid., 303.

70. Stewart et al., *Systematic Counseling*, 163.

71. Ibid., 164–170.

72. Ibid., 173–175.

73. Ibid., 176.

74. Patricia A. Wisocki and Edward Rooney, "A Comparison of Thought Stopping and Covert Sensitization Techniques in the Treatment of Smoking: A Brief Report," *The Psychological Record* 24 (1974): 192.

75. Cormier and Cormier, *Interviewing Strategies*, 342.

76. D.C. Rimm and J.C. Masters, *Behavior Therapy: Techniques and Empirical Findings* (New York: Academic Press, 1974), 416–449.

77. John Anthony and Barry A. Edelstein, "Thought Stopping Treatment of Anxiety Attacks Due to Seizure-Related Obsessive Ruminations," *Journal of Behavior Therapy and Experimental Psychiatry* 6 (1975): 343–344.

78. Louis Gershman, "Case Conference: A Transvestite Fantasy Treated by Thought Stopping, Covert Sensitization and Aversive Shock," *Journal of Behavior Therapy and Experimental Psychiatry* 1 (1970): 153–161.

79. Toshiko Yamagami, "The Treatment of an Obsession by Thought Stopping," *Journal of Behavior Therapy and Experimental Psychiatry* 2 (1971): 133–135.

80. Joseph Wolpe, "Dealing with Resistance to Thought Stopping: A Transcript," *Journal of Behavior Therapy and Experimental Psychiatry* 2 (1971): 121–125.

81. Michael J. Mahoney and Kathryn Mahoney, *Permanent Weight Control, A Total Solution of the Dieter's Dilemma* (New York: W.W. Norton & Company, 1976), 46–68.

82. Ibid., 65.

83. Ibid., 62–63.

84. Rimm and Masters, *Behavior Therapy*, 416–449.

85. Cormier and Cormier, *Interviewing Strategies*, 362–370.

86. B.F. Skinner, *Science and Human Behavior* (New York: The Free Press, 1965), 64–66, 72–75.

87. Albert Bandura, *Principles of Behavior Modification* (New York: Holt, Rinehart & Winston, 1969), 143–148.

88. Frederick H. Kanfer and Jeanne S. Phillips, *Learning Foundations of Behavior Therapy* (New York: John Wiley & Sons, 1970), 241–368.

89. Arthur R. Cohen, *Attitude Change and Social Influence* (New York: Basic Books, 1964), 129–140.

90. Kanfer and Phillips, *Learning Foundations*, 241–318.

91. Leonard P. Ullman and Leonard Krasner, *A Psychological Approach to Abnormal Behavior* (Englewood Cliffs, N.J.: Prentice-Hall, 1975), 224–247.

92. James G. Holland and B.F. Skinner, *Analysis of Behavior* (New York: McGraw-Hill Book Company, 1961), 98–105, 132–136.

93. Albert Bandura, *Principles of Behavior Modification* (New York: Holt, Rinehart & Winston, 1969), 182–202.

94. Holland and Skinner, *Analysis,* 118–131.

95. Sackett and Haynes, ed., *Compliance,* 110–118.

96. Marjorie E. Seybold and Daniel B. Drachman, "Gradually Increasing Doses of Prednisone in Myasthenia Gravis: Reducing the Hazards of Treatment," *New England Journal of Medicine* 290 (1974): 81–84.

97. Harold Leitenberg, ed., *Handbook of Behavior Modification and Behavior Therapy* (Englewood Cliffs, N.J.: Prentice-Hall, 1976), 440–441.

98. Sydnor B. Penick et al., "Behavior Modification in the Treatment of Obesity," *Psychosomatic Medicine* 33 (1971): 49–55.

99. T.F. Plant, "Doctor's Order and Patient Compliance: Letter to the Editor," *New England Journal of Medicine* 292 (1974): 435.

100. Sackett and Haynes, ed., *Compliance,* 100–109.

101. Stewart et al., *Systematic Counseling,* 208–209.

102. Ibid., 210.

103. Ibid., 211–214.

104. Ibid., 223.

105. Ibid., 224.

106. Ibid., 228–229.

107. Ibid., 230.

108. Ibid., 232.

109. Ibid.

110. Ibid., 232–234.

111. Ibid., 238.

112. Ibid., 239.

113. Ibid.

114. Ibid., 240.

115. Ibid., 240–241.

116. Ibid., 242.

117. Foods and Nutrition Resource Center, ed., *Counseling Manual,* 29.

118. Ibid.

119. Ibid.

120. J.P. Madden, S.J. Goodman, and H.A. Buthrie, "Validity of the 24-Hour Recall," *Journal of the American Dietetic Association* 68 (1976): 143–147.

121. Foods and Nutrition Resource Center, ed., *Counseling Manual,* 30.

122. B.R. Soutter and M.C. Kennedy, "Patient Compliance Assessment in Drug Trials: Usage and Methods," *Australian and New Zealand Journal of Medicine* 4 (1974): 360–364.

123. National Diet-Heart Study, "Final Report."

124. Foods and Nutrition Resource Center, ed., *Counseling Manual,* 30–31.

125. Rose Ann L. Shorey, Bennett Sewell, and Michael O'Brien, "Efficacy of Diet and Exercises in the Reduction of Serum Cholesterol and Triglycerides in Free Living Adult Males," *American Journal of Clinical Nutrition* 29 (1976): 512–521.

126. Sharron S. Coplin, Jean Hines, and Annette Gormican, "Outpatient Dietary Management of the Prader-Willi Syndrome," *Journal of the American Dietetic Association* 68 (1976): 330–334.

127. Research Committee, "Low-fat Diet in Myocardial Infarction: A Controlled Trial," *Lancet* 2 (1965): 501–504.

128. M.C. Burk and F.M. Pao, "Methodology for Large-Scale Surveys of Household and Individual Diets," *Home Economics Research Report,* no. 4.

129. Foods and Nutrition Resource Center, ed., *Counseling Manual,* 30–31.

130. Stewart et al., *Systematic Counseling,* 251–253.

Part II

Application of Interviewing and Counseling Skills

This part discusses problems with eating behaviors associated with certain prescribed dietary patterns involving modifications in calories, fat and cholesterol, carbohydrates, protein, sodium, and in bland foods. Each chapter is based on the following outline:

1. Common inappropriate eating behaviors associated with the diet
2. Assessing individual eating behaviors
3. Treatment strategies to combat inappropriate eating behaviors
   a. Behavioral strategies
   b. Cueing devices
   c. Nutrition basics
4. Evaluating new appropriate eating behaviors
   a. Monitoring devices
   b. Evaluation or checklists
      • Client
      • Counselor
5. Examples of dietary adherence tools
6. Reading list.

Initially each chapter discusses possible problem eating patterns, then reviews assessment techniques designed to determine individual behaviors that are inappropriate to the prescribed diet. Treatment of such inappropriate conduct is analyzed in terms of behavioral strategies, cueing devices, and nutrition concepts, ending with ways to monitor client progress. In each chapter, two checklists are provided: (1) on eating behavior for client and counselor use, and (2) for determining the counselor's effectiveness.

All of these elements need to be individualized for each client and, indeed, may be inappropriate for some individuals. Discussion of suggested assessment, treatment, and evaluation for specific dietary patterns should be encouraged if this book is used as a classroom text, since there are many alternatives to each problem.

Chapters 4 through 9 provide examples of two types of adherence tools: (1) that can be used as a monitoring device to determine how well the clients are adhering to their dietary patterns, and (2) that supplement the basic dietary instruction. The examples are designed with the following in mind:

1. The tool has a goal or an objective.
2. The tool gains the client's attention.
3. The tool is concise and to the point.
4. The tool makes allowances for individual differences in eating habits.

Figure II-1 Qualitative Rating of Counselor's Helping Style

	Rarely	Occasionally	Undecided	Often	Almost Always
1. Did the nutrition counselor appear to be comfortable with the client and with the subject areas discussed?					
2. Did the counselor avoid imposing values on the client?					
3. Did the counselor remain objective?					
4. Did the counselor focus on the client, not just on the procedure of providing a diet instruction?					
5. Were the counselor's skills spontaneous and nonmechanical?					
6. How would you describe the likelihood of the client's returning to this nutrition counselor again?					
Comments from Rater or Client					

Source: Adapted from *Interviewing Strategies for Helpers* by William H. Cormier and L. Sherilyn Cormier, published by Brooks/Cole Publishing Company, Monterey, Calif., pp. 112, 114. Copyright © 1979, by permission of Brooks/Cole Publishing Company.

Figure II-2 Quantitative Rating of Counselors

| Nutrition Counselor Statement No. | Verbal Responses — Listening | | | | | Action | | | Sharing | | Teaching | | | Nonverbal Behavior — Eyes | | Face | | Body | | | | | | Para-linguistics | | |
	Clarification	Paraphrase	Reflection of Feeling	Summarization	Probe	Ability Potential	Confrontation	Interpretation	Self-Disclosure	Immediacy	Instructions	Verbal Setting Operation	Information Giving	Initiates Eye Contact	Breaks Eye Contact	Head Nods	Smiles	Body Facing Client	Body Turned Away	Body Leaning Forward	Body Leaning Backward	Body Relaxed	Body Tense	Completed Sentences	Broken Sentences	Speech Errors
1																										
2																										
3																										
4																										
5																										
6																										
7																										
8																										
9																										
10																										
Total																										

Source: Adapted from *Interviewing Strategies for Helpers* by William H. Cormier and L. Sherilyn Cormier, published by Brooks/Cole Publishing Company, Monterey, Calif., p. 113. Copyright © 1979, by permission of Brooks/Cole Publishing Company.

Each chapter is followed by a reading list that should be used in conjunction with the text to ensure that appropriate nutrition practices, interviewing, and counseling are carried out together.

Each chapter also includes a review of the content; answers to the review questions appear in Appendix I.

Health professionals who do not have formal training in dietetics should work closely with a registered dietitian in recommending changes for special regimens. For example, the renal diet can include many complicated changes. Dietitians trained in that field should be consulted.

Figures II–1 and II–2 provide qualitative and quantitative evaluations of interviewing styles that can be used with each session and subject in the remaining chapters. They also can be used as a check to be sure basic skills have been acquired prior to beginning Part II.

Following are instructions for using these two rating instruments.

The quantitative scoring involves obtaining a frequency count of the types of the counselors' verbal and nonverbal responses. For each counselor statement, the type of verbal and nonverbal response should be indicated. At the end of the interview, the number of responses associated with each category are tallied.

The qualitative rating involves a subjective judgment by a rater or by the client (or both) about aspects of the counselor's style. After observing the interview for each of the six items, the appropriate box is checked to represent the rater/client's judgment about the counselor during most of the interview. Comments can be added at the bottom of the rating sheets.

Chapter 4

Counseling for Low-Calorie Eating Patterns

Objectives for Chapter 4

1. Identify common inappropriate behaviors associated with weight gain or overeating.
2. Identify steps in assessing individual eating behaviors.
3. Identify strategies to treat inappropriate eating behaviors contributing to weight gain.
4. Generate appropriate strategies to counsel overweight clients to control eating patterns.
5. Identify elements necessary for both client and counselor evaluation.
6. Recommend certain dietary adherence tools for weight-loss clients.

4

INAPPROPRIATE EATING BEHAVIORS

Which of these thought processes are associated with weight gain?

- "I deserve it."
- "It's just no use. I have no willpower."
- "I'm bored."
- "I'm off that rotten diet now."

Each of these can have a direct bearing on individuals' propensity to gain weight. Nutrition counselors must be aware of a variety of thought processes as well as overt eating behaviors before trying to assess the major problem. It always is important to try to identify antecedents and consequences of inappropriate eating behaviors.

Many present or future clients begin thinking about weight loss in terms of going on and off diets: "I go on a diet to lose weight. Usually I can't stand the diet. I just wait until I lose 10 or 15 pounds and then go back to eating those really good foods I'm accustomed to." This particular syndrome frequently is associated with alternating increases and decreases in weight.

Nutrition counselors might consider generally trying to avoid the term "diet" in their instructions to describe a means toward weight loss. The rationale is that along with the word "diet" the two negative words "going off" tend to follow.

Many clients will suggest that food is a kind of reward: "When I finish the housework (or reach the 3 P.M. break at my job) I feel like I deserve a reward so I just go to the refrigerator (or vending machines or cafeteria). Right there in front of me are all the rewards I need. I really deserve to eat in payment for my hard work."

Signals or cues to eat are everywhere. Counselors should study each client's environment and note specific cues that trigger inappropriate eating behaviors. At home, candy near the television set can trigger snacking responses that might not occur otherwise. TV commercials may provide stimulus to go to the kitchen for potato chips, candy bars, beverages, etc.

Many clients will admit that boredom can be a cause of inappropriate eating behaviors: "I eat because there is nothing else to do." Counselors can suggest many substitutes for eating to eliminate boredom and possibly increase activity. In some cases hobbies can serve as substitutes for eating, i.e., doing needlework or polishing shoes instead of snacking while watching TV.

Some inappropriate behaviors involve rapid eating. It appears as though the client is saying, "How fast can I clear this plate?" Along with this is the inability to listen when the body provides signals of fullness or satiety. Booth states that satiety may cease to originate solely from gastric motility and distention or a physiological state and that the power of suggestion also may play a large role in providing signals of fullness.[1]

In the eating chain syndrome as described by Ferguson,[2] activities can be used to break up patterns that lead to inappropriate behaviors. He says that eating occurs at one end of a chain of responses. If the counselors work backward from the terminal behavior of eating, events or cues in the environment that started the chain of events leading to it can be identified.

Much of what goes on in the client's head, such as negative thoughts, can trigger inappropriate eating behaviors. The client who is thinking, "I'm really a rotten person for eating that piece of candy. It's no use. I might as well eat myself sick," probably will overeat out of despair. Mahoney and Mahoney describe the reversal of this process as "cognitive ecology."[3] By substituting positive thoughts for negative ones, clients can develop a built-in self-reward system.

In some cases lack of exercise can be a problem. Some clients may complain, "I just don't feel like moving."

ASSESSMENT OF EATING BEHAVIORS

The nutrition counselors' next task is assessment of clients' eating behaviors. The first step is to try to identify the general problem from the many that may surface in a general interview. Overweight clients may not really want to lose weight but appear at a counseling session because their spouse or doctor has sent them. In some cases the major problem may be totally psychological and referral to a specialist in that field may be the best course of action.

If referral does not seem necessary, the next step is data collection. Six factors related to weight gain data should be emphasized.

1. eating patterns
2. food quantities
3. food quality
4. activity levels
5. food-related thoughts
6. food-related cues

Exhibit 4–1 presents instructions and a form to use in gathering information in each of these categories and Figure 4–1 a sample already filled out.

Other authors also discuss the vital importance of assessment for obese clients. Brownell states that these categories are important to cover:[4]

1. physiology
2. eating behaviors
3. physical activity
4. psychological and social adjustment.

Physiological factors can include an assessment of cell size and number. In assessing physical status, several categories should be considered: endocrine, hypothalmic, cardiopulmonary, orthopedic, genetic, weight, and family history. Bray and Teague provide an algorithm for the medical assessment of obese clients.[5] The steps necessary in diagnosing medical problems of an obese patient are delineated.

In the physiological analysis, counselors also should be concerned about body fat, which can be assessed through a variety of tests. The one most commonly used is skinfold thickness, using a caliper. Body weight is an indicator of physical status.

Eating behaviors are very important to eventual treatment. The most frequently used assessment method is a diet record. This can provide details on food preferences, eating style, environmental cues to eating, and amounts eaten.

Physical activity is an important component in any weight-loss program. Counselors should check on exercise during both working and nonworking hours. Equally important is psychological and social functioning. Psychological functioning can include positive and negative monologues as described earlier; social functioning deals with responses by spouse, children, coworkers, or friends to weight loss and eating behaviors.

Exhibit 4–1 Data Collection Chart

Instructions for Filling Out the Food Diary

Time: Starting time for a meal or snack

Minutes spent eating: Length of the eating episode in minutes

M/S: meal or snack: Indicate type of eating by the appropriate letter, "M" or "S"

H: Hunger on a scale of 0 to 3, with 0 = no hunger, 3 = extreme hunger

Body position:

  1. walking
  2. standing
  3. sitting
  4. lying down

Activity while eating: Record any activity you carry out while eating, such as watching television, reading, function in a workplace, or sweeping the floor.

Location of eating: Record each place you eat, such as your car, workplace, kitchen table, living room couch, or bed.

Food type and quantity: Indicate the content of your meal or snack by kind of food and quantity. Choose units of measurement that you will be able to reproduce from week to week. Accuracy is not as important as consistency.

Eating with whom: Indicate with whom you are eating or whether you are eating that meal or snack alone.

Feelings before and during eating: Record your feelings or mood immediately before (B) or while (W) eating. Typical feelings are angry, bored, confused, depressed, frustrated, sad, etc.

Minutes spent exercising today: Record the total number of minutes you spent exercising, followed by the type of exercise—walking, jogging, running, riding a bicycle or a horse, dancing, skiing, swimming, bowling, etc.

Day of Week_____   Name_____

Time	Minutes Spent Eating	M/S	H	Body Position	Activity While Eating	Location of Eating	Food Type and Quantity	Eating With Whom	Feeling Before (B) and while (W) Eating	Minutes Spent Exercising Today
6:00										
11:00										
4:00										

Exhibit 4-1 continued

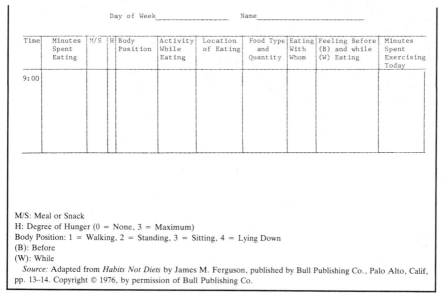

Day of Week_____   Name_____

Time	Minutes Spent Eating	M/S	H	Body Position	Activity While Eating	Location of Eating	Food Type and Quantity	Eating With Whom	Feeling Before (B) and while (W) Eating	Minutes Spent Exercising Today
9:00										

M/S: Meal or Snack
H: Degree of Hunger (0 = None, 3 = Maximum)
Body Position: 1 = Walking, 2 = Standing, 3 = Sitting, 4 = Lying Down
(B): Before
(W): While
    Source: Adapted from *Habits Not Diets* by James M. Ferguson, published by Bull Publishing Co., Palo Alto, Calif, pp. 13–14. Copyright © 1976, by permission of Bull Publishing Co.

TREATMENT STRATEGIES

In the third step nutrition counselors use the Food Diary Form in Exhibit 4-1 to identify a wealth of information related to eventual treatment. Assessment based on this form can lead to identification of causes of weight gain and of strategies to achieve and maintain ideal body weight.

Before selecting a strategy, the numerous alternative methods should be analyzed. Coates reviews various psychological strategies[6] and Stunkard studies several different methods of treating overweight clients.[7]

1. calorie counting
2. behavior modification
3. self-help groups, i.e., TOPS (Take Off Pounds Sensibly), Weight Watchers, Overeaters Anonymous etc.
4. jejunoileal and gastric bypass surgery
5. drugs to increase metabolic rate and suppress appetite
6. popular "lose pounds quick" diets.

The problems associated with the last three methods in the list also are presented.[8]

Figure 4–1 Example of a Completed Food Diary Form

SAMPLE

Day of Week __MONDAY__   Name __R.S.T.__

Time	Minutes Spent Eating	M/S	H	Body Position	Activity While Eating	Location of Eating	Food Type and Quantity	Eating With Whom	Feeling Before (B) and while (W) Eating	Minutes Spent Exercising Today
6:00 7:20-30	10 min	M	0	3	PAPER	KITCHEN	8oz. Coffee 1 cup cereal	WIFE	HAPPY	40 minutes
8:15-20	5 min	S	0	2	TALKING	WORK	4oz wholemilk 1 cal-doughnut 8oz. coffee	FRIENDS	TIRED (B)	WALKING
10:30?	5 min	S	1	1	WALKING	HALL	1 cake doughnut	ALONE	LATE (W)	
11:00										
12:30	1 min	S	2	2	WORK	DESK	1-1.5oz Snicker	ALONE	LATE (W)	
3:30- 3:40	10 min	M	3	3	READING	RESTAURANT	1-8oz Coke 3oz ckd. hamburger patty 1 Hamb. Bun	ALONE	TIRED (B)	
4:00 5:30- 6:00	30 min.	S	3	3	Paper TV	L.R.	1oz SCOTCH 1/4 cup peanuts	FAMILY	TIRED (B)	
6:00- 7:00	1 hour	M	2	3	TV	D.R.	Beef TV Dinner 1 cup ice cream	FAMILY	ANGRY (B)	
9:00										
10:30- 10:45	15 min	S	0	2	TV	L.R.	1/2 cup ice cream	WIFE	BORED (B)	

M/S: Meal or Snack
H: Degree of Hunger (0 = None, 3 = Maximum)
Body Position: 1 = Walking, 2 = Standing, 3 = Sitting, 4 = Lying Down
(B): Before
(W): While
  Source: Adapted from *Habits Not Diets* by James M. Ferguson, published by Bull Publishing Co., Palo Alto, Calif., pp. 13–14. Copyright © 1976, by permission of Bull Publishing Co.

No one strategy will be fully effective for all clients; rather, in many cases, a combination may be the answer. It is important to remember that each client has a problem that is unique and may require a helping strategy unlike that used with the previous person.

After the strategy has been selected is the time to begin experimenting and collecting data. Baseline data should be compared with information collected during strategy implementation. Once a strategy has been adopted, it should be modified when necessary.

What are some strategies to combat inappropriate eating behaviors? One is substitution of nonfood-related activities. With this method, it is necessary to work with the clients in developing a list of enjoyable activities, particularly those requiring substantial expenditure of energy. The information obtained in the Data Collection Chart (Exhibit 4–1, supra) can suggest a starting point.

It is preferable to select activities that fit into the clients' daily routine, based on their suggestions as to which ones would work best. This is a time when counselors' listening skills and encouragement for the clients can generate solutions that will lead to optimum results. Instead of eating, clients can turn to substitute activities such as those in Exhibit 4–2.

Interposing time between eating episodes is a second method for diminishing the urge. This strategy may require the use of a cooking timer, alarm clock, etc. Clients are asked to delay a snack for a certain number of minutes. Gradually they will be able to increase the time lapse between

---

Exhibit 4–2 Activity Substitutes for Eating

Clients can resort to numerous activities as alternates to overeating. They can:
- Rearrange furniture
- Spend extra time with a friend
- Play cards or a game with someone—chess, Monopoly, bridge, etc.
- Go to a movie, play, or concert
- Do something for charity
- Go to a museum
- Take a quiet walk
- Take a long, leisurely bubble bath
- Balance their checkbook
- Write a letter
- Make a phone call to a friend or relative
- Wash their hair
- Start a garden
- Do home repairs
- Write a creative poem or story
- Do some sewing or creative stitchery
- Do a crossword puzzle
- Go jogging
- Play golf
- Join a softball team
- Jump rope
- Take up weight lifting
- Go hiking
- Take up, or increase participation in, a sport.

the urge to snack and the actual act of eating to 10 or 15 minutes. During this interlude they should be encouraged to perform some other activity. They usually are amazed at how well this strategy curbs their appetites.

The third strategy is cue elimination. Exhibit 4–1 (supra) can help in determining which cues lead to improper eating. For example, by looking at a rough house plan and identifying where eating episodes are occurring, clients can set up roadblocks to those cues. Many clients will find their snacking locations show up in clusters around the television set, favorite chairs, or in the kitchen by the refrigerator or sink (or the cafeteria or vending machines at work). They may be shocked to find they eat in more places than they believed.

Ferguson has designed an exercise to help eliminate eating cues.[9]

1. Ask the clients to select a specific room in the house in which all eating should occur. This place should be regarded as relatively comfortable. They also should designate eating places away from home, such as in a restaurant, cafeteria, lunchroom, or by vending machines. They should be cautioned to avoid eating while working. This will break the chain of association between eating and other activities. It could be suggested that every designated eating place be special. If eating must occur with work, if at all feasible a place mat and silverware should be set, with a real (not plastic) cup for coffee or tea. At home, candlelight, flowers, attractive plates and silverware can make the designated place "special."

2. Ask the clients to change their usual eating place at the table. If, for example, it is the head, they should move to one side; if at the side, change with someone on the other side. The rationale is to break longstanding cues at the table.

3. Ask the clients to separate eating from other activities—to avoid combining eating with telephone conversations, watching TV, reading, working, etc. The emphasis should be on food with others and on making eating enjoyable by focusing on the taste and texture of the ingredients.

4. Ask clients to remove food from all places (particularly visible ones) except appropriate storage areas in the kitchen and to keep stored food out of sight by placing it in cupboards, in opaque containers, or in the refrigerator.

5. Suggest that clients keep fresh fruits and vegetables for snacks in attractive containers.

6. Request that they remove serving containers from the table during mealtimes.

Once the nutrition counselors have helped clients eliminate cues, the strategy can turn to slowly decreasing serving size. The use of smaller plates and smaller portions will decrease total caloric consumption. Nouvelle cuisine, with its very small portions arranged artistically in the center of large plates, is an attractive alternative. The foods need not involve fancy French cooking; the regular "menu" can simply be restaged in a fancier setting at no additional cost.

Many of these strategies involve getting help from spouse, family, and/or friends. The clients should be told to explain the strategies to anyone seen regularly. Closest friends' understanding of the program rationale can provide moral support. Through teaching others, the clients may grasp strategies more clearly.

Another strategy involves thinking positively. Appendix F gives examples of ways in which recordkeeping can help uncover negative thoughts associated with inappropriate eating behaviors. Getting clients to see how often negative thoughts force excessive food consumption can be a first step to weight control. This change from negative to positive thinking is very much an activity in which the clients are in charge. Counselors can provide examples of thoughts such as: "I'm such a failure. I can't do anything right. I might as well give up. Who cares if I stuff myself with this cake?"

This negative monologue with self can be transformed to more positive thinking: "I ate one piece of cake and even though it is high in calories I can stop with that one piece. I'm really feeling good about being able to stop without going ahead and eating the entire cake."

From that point on, the clients can formulate positive self-thoughts to replace their negative ones.

For most people, increasing exercise in combination with decreasing calories is helpful. Again Exhibit 4–1 is used to determine baseline activity levels. Many of the suggestions listed as substitutes for eating in Exhibit 4–2 (supra) involve an increase in activity. Counselors should encourage clients to enroll in exercise programs but caution any with physical or medical problems to check with a physician first.

Underlying all of these suggestions is a good nutrition base. Government authorities such as the U.S. Committee on Recommended Dietary Allowances (RDA) and the Canadian Ministry of Health and Welfare have published recommended energy intakes for various groups by age and sex.[10] The energy RDA meets the needs of an average person. It must be kept in mind that an energy deficit of 3,500 calories is necessary for the loss of a pound of body fat. This means that with a deficit of 500 calories per day, a pound of weight will be lost each week. Whitney and Hamilton find that the loss of more than two pounds of body fat a week rarely can be maintained.[11] They also caution that a diet supplying less than 1,200 calories per day can be made adequate in vitamins and minerals only with great difficulty.

To promote adequate nutrition, attention must be paid to nutrient levels. For adults, the recommended dietary allowances are .8 grams per kilogram of body weight per day.[12] For a 70-kilogram man, that would be 56 grams of protein per day, and for a 55-kilogram woman, 44 grams.

There is considerable difference of opinion as to whether carbohydrates or fats should be reduced in an energy-restricted diet. Significant weight reductions on carbohydrate-free diets probably result from loss of water bound to glycogen. Without carbohydrates in the diet, the body uses stored glycogen to maintain normal blood glucose levels. The water with its electrolytes that are bound to the glycogen is excreted by the kidneys.

An energy-restricted diet should provide vitamins and minerals at least equivalent to the Recommended Dietary Allowances. If calorie intake is very restricted (fewer than 1,000), vitamin and mineral supplements may be needed.

The alcohol content of the diet should be assessed carefully at baseline, particularly because clients tend to underestimate consumption. One gram of alcohol provides seven calories. Beer and wines contain carbohydrates that also contribute calories. The calories from alcoholic beverages may be the difference between losing and not losing weight.

Water and other nonnutritive fluids are not restricted unless there are heart or kidney complications.

Other approaches to weight loss are not covered here. However, the reading list that follows this chapter identifies numerous books that cover the use of exchange lists for weight reduction, starvation regimens, formula diets, anorexigenic agents, hormones, diuretics, laxatives, and ileal bypass surgery.

EVALUATION OF BEHAVIORS

Client progress is evaluated by comparing current and past data, as in Figure 4–2. Clients can be asked to extend a strategy, possibly by increasing negative-to-positive thought transformations. If a strategy is not working, it should be revised. For example, if finding a designated eating place at work poses problems, the nutrition counselor may need to discuss other means of cue elimination—using a place mat, plate, and silverware. In some cases, a new strategy may be appropriate. If clients find it impossible to substitute noneating activities for routine snacking, it may be necessary first to work to eliminate negative monologues, then add other activities as monologues are transformed to a more positive mode.

Figure 4–2 Diet Maintenance Data Collection

Day of Week _____ Name _____				
Time	*M/S*	*H*	*Food Type and Quantity*	*Minutes Spent Exercising and Type of Exercise*
6:00 a.m.				
11:00 a.m.				
4:00 p.m.				
9:00 p.m.				

M/S: Meal or Snack
H: Degree of Hunger (0 = none; 3 = maximum)

Source: Adapted from *Habits Not Diets* by James M. Ferguson, published by Bull Publishing Co., Palo Alto, Calif., p. 87. Copyright © 1976, by permission of Bull Publishing Co.

Exhibit 4–3 Client Checklist for Weight Control

_____ 1. My major goal was reached in solving the designated problem.
_____ 2. My eating patterns have changed.
_____ 3. My food quantities have changed.
_____ 4. My food quality has changed.
_____ 5. My activity level has increased.
_____ 6. My food-related thoughts are more positive.
_____ 7. I have eliminated most of the cues that formerly triggered inappropriate eating behaviors.

The clients can be asked to set up a checklist to determine how well the eating behavior changes are working. (Exhibit 4–3) The general checklist is geared toward looking at changes in behaviors associated with weight gain; nutrition counselors should work out a more specific one based on each individual client's problem.

The counselors' checklist (Exhibit 4–4) provides help in reviewing the success of the interview from the practitioners' viewpoint. This also might be made more specific for each client. In any case, the checklist should be set up in the manner most useful to each individual counselor.

Exhibit 4–4 Counselor Checklist for Weight Control Client

_____ 1. Did the counseling session address the client's major problem?
_____ 2. Did the client's goal appear to have been achieved?
_____ 3. Were the strategies for altering eating behaviors carried out efficiently?
_____ 4. Did I use appropriate verbal and nonverbal interviewing skills?
_____ 5. Where might changes have been made?

_____

_____

_____

_____ 6. Did I use appropriate counseling skills? _____
_____ 7. Where might changes have been made?

_____

_____

_____

_____ 8. What general changes would I make in the next counseling interview with a similar weight-loss client?

_____

_____

_____

_____

Now is the time to try putting the ideas in this chapter to use. The following are two situations involving weight-loss clients:

1. Jan, a 30-year-old female, is nearly 20 pounds overweight. She is very upset over this and has tried many ways toward quick and easy weight control—diet pills, fasting, fad diets, etc. Jan has a family of four and works from 8 a.m. to 5 p.m. at a dress shop. She prepares breakfast for her family each morning, eats at a cafeteria for lunch, and fixes dinner for the family each evening. Her major problem, she indicates, is evening snacking.

2. Dan, a 40-year-old male, is 30 pounds overweight. He frequently is depressed over his weight and has tried many lose-weight-quick treatments. All have failed. He lives alone and works nights on a line in a factory. He sleeps during the day and eats all of his meals away from home.

The nutrition counselors' assignment is to map out a plan for weight control in these clients using ideas discussed in this chapter and being sure to include assessment, treatment, and evaluation phases. A brief rationale for the strategy is to be written at the end of each plan.

Adherence Tool 4–1 Monitoring Device

Goal Attainment Chart

Suggestions:

Date _____

Goal: _____

Number of times I will achieve this goal: _____
Behavior Monitored: _____

	Days						
	1	2	3	4	5	6	7
If Did→ ☆							
If Did Not→ √							
Number of ☆s = _____							
Number of √s = _____							

Source: Nancy L. Schwartz, R.D.

Review of Chapter 4

(Answers in Appendix I)

1. In the following examples, identify the inappropriate eating behaviors associated with weight gain:

"I have followed this diet so religiously. I'm really proud of myself. The agony of passing up cocktails and opting for the diet drink at a party, the embarrassment of refusing my friend's seven-layer torte, the pain of refusing the birthday cake my kids made especially for me, and on and on. Those days are behind me now. I lost 20 pounds and now I'm home free."

Adherence Tool 4–2 Informational Device

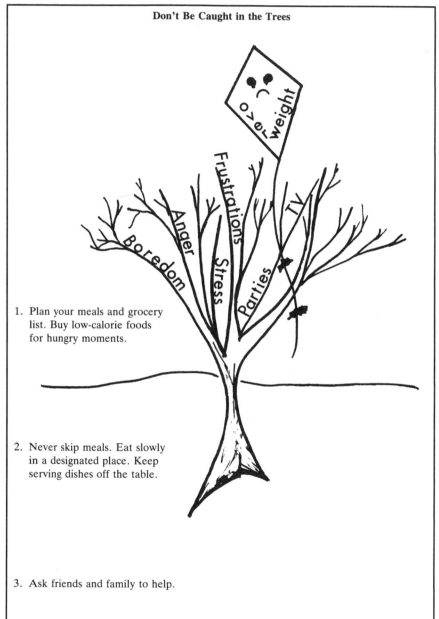

Don't Be Caught in the Trees

1. Plan your meals and grocery list. Buy low-calorie foods for hungry moments.

2. Never skip meals. Eat slowly in a designated place. Keep serving dishes off the table.

3. Ask friends and family to help.

Adherence Tool 4–2 continued

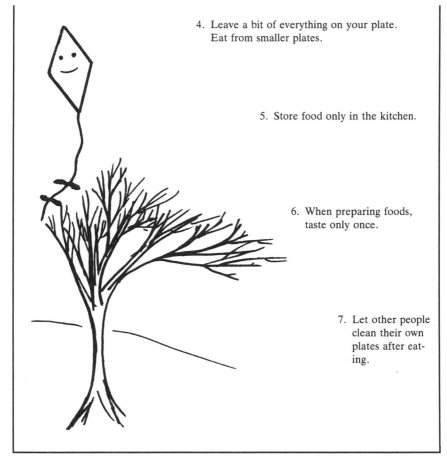

4. Leave a bit of everything on your plate. Eat from smaller plates.

5. Store food only in the kitchen.

6. When preparing foods, taste only once.

7. Let other people clean their own plates after eating.

What syndrome is this sort of thinking leading to?_____

"What is wrong with me? Don't I have any willpower? I look like a fat slob and yet I continue to eat. I'm just a hopeless case."

What syndrome does this sort of self-talk tell you as a counselor that the client is struggling with?_____

2. List three steps in assessing individual eating behaviors.

   a. _____

   b. _____

   c. _____

3. List six strategies that might be used to facilitate a client's weight loss.
    a. _____
    b. _____
    c. _____
    d. _____
    e. _____
    f. _____

4. Describe one situation in which you would use one or more of those six strategies. Indicate your rationale. _____
    _____
    _____
    _____

5. Identify seven possible questions to raise in evaluating client progress.
    a. _____
    b. _____
    c. _____
    d. _____
    e. _____
    f. _____
    g. _____

6. Identify six possible questions to review in evaluating your interviewing and counseling skills following a session with a client.
    a. _____
    b. _____
    c. _____
    d. _____
    e. _____
    f. _____

NOTES

1. David A. Booth, "Acquired Behavior Controlling Energy Input and Output," in Albert J. Stunkard, ed. *Obesity* (Philadelphia: W.B. Saunders Company, 1980), 102.

2. James M. Ferguson, *Habits Not Diets* (Palo Alto, Calif.: Bull Publishing Co., 1976), 65.

3. Michael J. Mahoney and Kathryn Mahoney, *Permanent Weight Control* (New York: W.W. Norton & Company, 1976), 46–68.

4. Kelly D. Brownell, "Assessment of Eating Disorders" in David Barlow, ed. Behavioral Assessment of Adult Disorders (New York: The Guilford Press, 1981), 366–374.

5. George Bray and R.J. Teague, "An Algorithm for the Medical Evaluation of Obese Patients" in Albert J. Stunkard, ed. *Obesity* (Philadelphia: W.B. Saunders Company, 1980).

6. Thomas J. Coates, "Eating—A Psychological Dilemma," *Journal of Nutrition Education* 13 (1981), Supplement, S34–S48.

7. Stunkard, *Obesity,* 249–394.

8. Ibid.

9. Ferguson, *Habits,* 31–32.

10. Food and Nutrition Board, *Recommended Dietary Allownces*, 9th ed. (Washington, D.C.: National Academy of Sciences, National Research Council, 1980), 186.

11. Eleanor Noss Whitney and Eva May Nunnelley Hamilton, *Understanding Nutrition* (St. Paul, Minn.: West Publishing Company, 1981), 248.

12. Food and Nutrition Board, *Recommended Dietary Allowances*, 46.

SUGGESTED READINGS
Books

Abramson, Edward E. *Behavioral Approaches to Weight Control.* New York: Springer Publishing Company, 1977.

American Dietetic Association. *Handbook of Clinical Dietetics.* New Haven, Conn.: Yale University Press, 1981.

Barlow, David, ed. *Behavioral Assessment of Adult Disorders* (Chap. 11, "Assessment of Eating Disorders"). New York: The Guilford Press, 1981.

Bray, George A. *The Obese Patient.* Philadelphia: W.B. Saunders Company, 1976.

Brownell, Kelly D. *Behavior Therapy for Weight Control: A Treatment Manual.* Philadelphia: K. D. Brownell, 1979.

Collipp, Platon J. *Childhood Obesity.* Littleton, Mass.: PSG Publishing Company, 1980.

Ferguson, James M. *Habits Not Diets.* Palo Alto, Calif.: Bull Publishing Co., 1976.

Foreyt, John Paul, ed. *Behavioral Treatments of Obesity.* New York: Pergamon Press, 1977.

Garrow, J.S. *Energy Balance and Obesity in Man.* New York: Elsevier, 1974.

Howard, A., ed. *Recent Advances in Obesity Research: I, Proceedings of the 1st International Congress on Obesity.* London: Newman Publishing, 1975.

Krause, Marie V., and Mahan, L. Kathleen. *Food, Nutrition and Diet Therapy.* Philadelphia: W. B. Saunders Company, 1979.

Mahoney, Michael J., and Mahoney, Kathryn. *Permanent Weight Control.* New York: W.W. Norton & Company, 1976.

Mitchell, Helen S. *Nutrition in Health and Disease.* Philadelphia: J.B. Lippincott Company, 1976.

Munro, J.F., ed. *The Treatment of Obesity.* Lancaster, England: MTP Press, 1979.

Powers, Pauline S. *Obesity, The Regulation of Weight.* Baltimore: The Williams and Wilkins Co., 1980.

Smith, Anne, ed. *Obesity, A Bibliography, 1974–1979.* London: Information Retrieval, Ltd., 1980.

Stuart, R.B. and Davis, B. *Slim Chance in a Fat World.* Champaign, Ill.: Research Press Co., 1978.

Stunkard, Albert J., ed. *Obesity.* Philadelphia: W.B. Saunders Company, 1980.

Articles

I. Behavioral Modification Treatments

Adams, Nancy. "The Eating Behavior of Obese and Non-Obese Women." *Behaviour Research and Therapy* 16(1978):225–232.

Beneke, William M., and Paulsen, Barbara K. "Long-term Efficacy of a Behavior Modification Weight Loss Program: A Comparison of Two Follow-up Maintenance Strategies." *Behavior Therapy* 10(1979):8–13.

Brownell, Kelly D., and Kaye, Frederick S. "A School-Based Behavior Modification, Nutrition Education, and Physical Activity Program for Obese Children." *American Journal of Clinical Nutrition* 35(1982):277–283.

Brownell, Kelly D., and Stunkard, Albert J. "Behavior Therapy and Behavior Change: Uncertainties in Programs for Weight Control." *Behaviour Research and Therapy* 16(1978):301.

Dunkel, L. Darrell, and Glaros, Alan G. "Comparison of Self-Instructional and Stimulus Control Treatments for Obesity." *Cognitive Therapy and Research* 2(1978):75–78.

Epstein, Leonard H., and Martin, John E. "Compliance and Side Effects of Weight Reduction Groups." *Behavior Modification* 1(1977):551–558.

Green, Leon. "Temporal and Stimulus Factors in Self-Monitoring by Obese Persons." *Behavior Therapy* 9(1978):328–341.

Grinker, Joel. "Behavioral and Metabolic Consequences of Weight Reduction." *Journal of the American Dietetic Association* 62(1973):30–34.

Hagen, Richard L.; Foreyt, John P.; and Durham, Thomas W. "The Dropout Problem: Reducing Attrition in Obesity Research." *Behavior Therapy* 7(1976):463–471.

Hall, Sharon M.; Bass, Anthony; and Monroe, James. "Continued Contact and Monitoring as Follow-Up Strategies: A Long-term Study of Obesity Treatment." *Addictive Behaviors* 3(1978):139–147.

Hall, Sharon M. "Follow-up Strategies in the Behavioral Treatment of Overweight." *Behaviour Research and Therapy* 13(1975):167–172.

Hanson, Richard W. "Use of Programmed Instruction in Teaching Self-Management Skills to Overweight Adults." *Behavior Therapy* 7(1976):366–373.

Herman, C. Peter, and Mack, Deborah. "Restrained and Unrestrained Eating." *Journal of Personality* 43(1975):647–660.

Herman, C. Peter; Polivy, Janet; and Silver, Roxanne. "The Effects of an Observer on Eating Behavior: The Induction of Sensible Eating." *Journal of Personality* 47(1979):85–99.

Jeffery, Robert W.; Thompson, P.D.; and Wing, Rena R. "Effects on Weight Reduction of Strong Monetary Contracts for Caloric Restriction or Weight Loss." *Behaviour Research and Therapy* 16(1978):363–370.

Jeffery, Robert W.; Wing, Rena R.; and Stunkard, Albert J. "Behavioral Treatment of Obesity: The State of the Art." *Behavior Therapy* 9(1978):189–199.

Johnson, William G. "The Development and Evaluation of a Behavioral Weight-Reduction Program." *International Journal of Obesity* 3(1979):229–238.

Jordon, Henry A., and Levitz, Leonard S. "Behavior Modification in a Self-Help Group." *Journal of the American Dietetic Association* 62(1973):27–29.

Kingsley, Raymond E. "Set-Points and Body-Weight Regulation ." *Psychiatric Clinical Nutrition of America* 1(1978):523–533.

Kingsley, Raymond G., and Wilson, G. Terrance. "Behavior Therapy for Obesity: A Comparative Investigation of Long-Term Efficacy." *Journal of Consulting and Clinical Psychology* 45(1977):288–298.

Kissileff, K.S.; Jordon, H.H.; and Levitz, L.S. "Eating Habits of Obese and Normal Weight Humans." *International Journal of Obesity* 2(1978):379.

Kristein, Marvin M.; Arnold, Charles B.; and Wynder, Ernst L. "Health Economics and Preventive Care." *Science* 195(1977):457–462.

Levitz, Leonard S., and Stunkard, Albert J. "A Therapeutic Coalition for Obesity: Behavior Modification and Patient Self-Help." *American Journal of Psychiatry* 131(1974):423–427.

Loro, Albert D. Jr.; Fisher E.B. Jr.; and Levenkron, Jeffrey C. "Comparison of Established and Innovative Weight-Reduction Treatment Procedures." *Journal of Applied Behavior Analysis* 12(1979):141–155.

Mahoney, Michael J. "Self-Reward and Self-Monitoring Techniques for Weight Control." *Behavior Therapy* 5(1974):48–57.

————. "Fat Fiction." *Behavior Therapy* 6(1975):416–418.

————. "Behavior Modification in the Treatment of Obesity." *Psychiatric Clinics of North America* 1(1978):651–660.

Mann, Ronald A. "The Behavior-Therapeutic Use of Contingency Contracting to Control an Adult Behavior Problem: Weight Control." *Journal of Applied Behavior Analysis* 5(1972):99–109.

McKenna, Ralph J. "Some Effects of Anxiety Level and Food Cues on the Eating Behavior of Obese and Normal Subjects." *Journal of Personality and Social Psychology* 22(1972):311–319.

Nisbett, Richard. "Hunger, Obesity, and the Ventromedial Hypothalamus." *Psychological Review* 79(1972):433–470.

Ohlson, Margaret A., and Harper, Laura Jane. "Longitudinal Studies of Food Intake and Weight of Women from Ages 18 to 56 Years." *Journal of the American Dietetic Association* 69(1976):626–631.

Öst, Lars-Göran, and Götestam, K. Gunnar. "Behavioral and Pharmacological Treatments for Obesity: An Experimental Comparison." *Addictive Behaviors* 1(1976):331–338.

Penick, Sydnor. "Behavior Modification in the Treatment of Obesity." *Psychosomatic Medicine* 33(1971):49–55.

Polivy, Janet. "Perception of Calories and Regulation of Intake in Restrained and Unrestrained Subjects." *Addictive Behaviors* 1(1976):237–244.

Rodin, Judith. "Environmental Factors in Obesity." *Psychiatric Clinics of North America* 1(1978):581–592.

Rosenthal, Barbara S., and Marx, Robert D. "Differences in Eating Patterns of Successful and Unsuccessful Dieters, Untreated Overweight and Normal Weight Individuals." *Addictive Behaviors* 3(1978):129–134.

Rush, Augustus J. "Comparative Efficacy of Cognitive Therapy and Pharmacotherapy in the Treatment of Depressed Outpatients." *Cognitive Therapy and Research* 1(1977):17–37.

Stalonas, Peter M.; Johnson, William G.; and Christ, Mary Ann. "Behavior Modification for Obesity: The Evaluation of Exercise, Contingency Management and Program Adherence." *Journal of Consulting and Clinical Psychology*. 46(1978):463–469.

Stuart, Richard B., and Guire, Kenneth. "Some Correlates of the Maintenance of Weight Loss Through Behavior Modification." *International Journal of Obesity* 2(1978):225–235.

Stuart, Richard B., and Mitchell, Christine. "A Professional and a Consumer Perspective on Self-Help Weight Control Groups." *Psychiatric Clinics of North America* 1(1978):697–712.

Stunkard, Albert J. "Basic Mechanisms Which Regulate Body Weight. New Perspectives." *Psychiatric Clinics of North America* 1(1978):461–472.

———. "Behavioral Treatment of Obesity: The Current Status." *International Journal of Obesity* 2(1978):237–249.

Stunkard, Albert J., and Kaplan D. "Eating in Public Places: A Review of Reports of the Direct Observation of Eating Behavior." *International Journal of Obesity* 1(1977):89–101.

Stunkard, Albert J., and Penick, Sydnor. "Behavior Modification in the Treatment of Obesity: The Problem of Maintaining Weight Loss." *Archives of General Psychiatry* 36(1979):801–806.

Taylor, C. Barr; Ferguson, James M.; and Reading, James C. "Gradual Weight Loss and Depression" *Behavior Therapy* 9(1978):622–625.

Van Itallie, Theodore B. "Dietary Fiber and Obesity." *American Journal of Clinical Nutrition* 31(1978):543–552.

———. "Diets for Weight Reduction; Mechanisms of Action and Physiological Effects." *International Journal of Obesity* 2(1978):113–122.

Waxman, Marjorie, and Stunkard, Albert J. "Caloric Intake and Expenditure of Obese Boys." *Journal of Pediatrics* 96(1980)187–193.

Williams, A.E., and Duncan, B.A. "A Commercial Weight-Reducing Organization: A Critical Analysis." *The Medical Journal of Australia* 1(1976):781–785.

———. "Comparative Results of an Obesity Clinic and a Commercial Weight Reducing Organization." *The Medical Journal of Australia* 1(1976):800–802.

Wilson, G. Terrance. "Methodological Considerations in Treatment Outcome Research on Obesity." *Journal of Consulting and Clinical Psychology* 46(1978):687–702.

Wollersheim, Janet P. "Effectiveness of Group Therapy Based Upon Learning Principles in the Treatment of Overweight Women." *Journal of Abnormal Psychology* 76(1970):462–474.

Wooley, Susan C.; Wooley, Orland W.; and Dyrenforth, Susan R. "Theoretical, Practical, and Social Issues in Behavioral Treatments of Obesity." *Journal of Applied Behavior Analysis* 12(1979):3–26.

Yates, Brian T. "Improving the Cost/Effectiveness of Obesity Programs: Three Basic Strategies for Reducing Cost Per Pound." *International Journal of Obesity* 2(1978):249–267.

II. Social Environment

Brownell, Kelly D. "The Effect of Couples Training and Partner Cooperativeness in the Behavioral Treatment of Obesity." *Behaviour Research and Therapy* 16(1978):323–333.

Cobb, Sidney. "Social Support As a Moderator of Life Stress." *Psychosomatic Medicine* 38(1976):300–314.

Goldblatt, Phillip B.; Moore, Mary E.; and Stunkard, Albert J. "Social Factors in Obesity." *Journal of the American Medical Association* 192(1965):1039–1044.

Levitz, Leonard, and Stunkard, Albert J. "A Therapeutic Coalition for Obesity: Behavior Modification and Patient Self-Help." *American Journal of Psychiatry* 131(1974):423–427.

Stunkard, Albert J. "From Explanation to Action in Psychosomatic Medicine: The Case of Obesity." *Psychosomatic Medicine* 37(1975):195–236.

Wilson, G. Terrance, and Brownell, Kelly D. "Behavior Therapy for Obesity: Including Family Members in the Treatment Process." *Behavior Therapy* 9(1978):943–945.

III. Positive Thinking

Garrow, J.S., and Stalley, Susan. "Cognitive Thresholds and Human Body Weight." *Proceeding of the Nutrition Society* 36(1977):18A.

Kirsch, Irving. "The Placebo Effect and the Cognitive-Behavioral Revolution." *Cognitive Therapy and Research* 2(1978):255–264.

Porikos, Katherine P., Booth, Glenn, and Van Itallie, Theodore B. "Effect of Covert Nutritive Dilution on Spontaneous Food Intake of Obese Individuals: A Pilot Study." *American Journal of Clinical Nutrition* 30(1977):1638–1644.

Slochower, Joyce. "Emotional Labeling and Overeating in Obese and Normal Weight Individuals." *Psychosomatic Medicine* 38(1976):131–139.

IV. Physical Activity

Apfelbaum, Mariam; Bostsarron, Jean; and Lacatis, D. "Effect of Caloric Restriction and Excessive Caloric Intake on Energy Expenditure." *American Journal of Clinical Nutrition* 24(1971):1405–1409.

Björntorp, Per. "Exercise and Obesity." *Psychiatric Clinics of North America* 1(1978):691–696.

Björntorp, Per. "Physical Training in Human Obesity. III. Effects of Long-term Physical Training on Body Composition." *Metabolism* 22(1973):1467–1475.

Björntorp, Per. "Physical Training in Human Hyperplastic Obesity, IV. Effects on Hormonal Status." *Metabolism* 26(1977):319–328.

Boyle, P.C.; Storlien, H.L.; and Keesey, R.E. "Increased Efficiency of Food Utilization Following Weight Loss." *Physiology and Behavior* 21(1978):261–264.

Brownell, Kelly D.; Stunkard, Albert J.; and Albaum, Janet Michelle. "Evaluation and Modification of Activity Patterns in the Natural Environment." *American Journal of Psychiatry* 137(1980):1540–1545.

Bullen, Beverly A.; Reed, Robert B.; and Mayer, Jean. "Physical Activity of Obese and Nonobese Adolescent Girls Appraised by Motion Picture Sampling." *American Journal of Clinical Nutrition* 14(1964):211–233.

Buskirk, E.R. "Obesity: A Brief Overview with Emphasis on Exercise." *Federation Proceedings* 33(1974):1948–1951.

Dahlkoetter, Jo Ann; Callahan, Edward J.; and Linton, John. "Obesity and the Unbalanced Energy Equation: Exercise vs. Eating Habit Change." *Journal of Consulting and Clinical Psychology* 47(1979):898–905.

Duddleston, Anne K., and Bennion, Marion. "Effect of Diet and/or Exercise on Obese College Women." *Journal of the American Dietetic Association* 56(1970):126–129.

Epstein, Leonard H., and Wing, Rena R. "Prescribed Level of Caloric Restriction in Behavioral Weight Loss Programs." *Addictive Behaviors* 6(1981):139–144.

Epstein, Leonard H.; Wing Rena R.; and Thompson, J. Kevin. "The Relationship Between Exercise Intensity, Caloric Intake and Weight." *Addictive Behaviors* 3(1978):185–190.

Gettman, Larry R.; Pollock, Michael L.; and Durstine, J. Larry. "Physiological Responses of Men to 1, 3, and 5 Day Per Week Training Programs." *Research Quarterly* 47(1976):638–646.

Gwinup, Grant, "Effect of Exercise Alone on the Weight of Obese Women." *Archives of Internal Medicine* 135(1975):676–680.

Krotkiewski, M.; Sjöstrom, L.; and Sullivan, L. "Effects of Long-Term Training on Adipose Tissue Cellularity and Body Composition in Hypertrophic and Hyperplastic Obesity." *International Journal of Obesity* 2(1978):395.

Maxfield, E., and Konishi, F. "Patterns of Food Intake and Physical Activity in Obesity." *Journal of the American Medical Association* 49(1966):406–408.

Ravussin, Eric. "Twenty-four-hour Energy Expenditure and Resting Metabolic Rate in Obese, Moderately Obese, and Control Subjects." *American Journal of Clinical Nutrition* 35(1982):566–573.

Schutz, Y. "Spontaneous Physical Activity Measured by Radar in Obese and Control Subjects Studied in a Respiration Chamber." *International Journal of Obesity* 6(1982):23–28.

Sheldahl, Lois M. "Effects of Exercise in Cool Water on Body Weight Loss." *International Journal of Obesity* 4(1982):29–42.

Stalonas, Peter M.; Johnson, William G.; Christ, Maryann. "Behavior Modification for Obesity: The Evaluation of Exercise, Contingency Management, and Program Adherence." *Journal of Consultation and Clinical Psychology* 46(1978):463–469.

Waxman, Marjorie, and Stunkard, Albert J. "Caloric Intake and Expenditure of Obese Children." *Journal of Pediatrics* 96(1980):187–193.

V. Nutrition Principles and Studies

Bistrian, Bruce R.; Blackburn, George L.; Flatt, Jean-Pierre; "Nitrogen Metabolism and Insulin Requirements in Obese Adults on a Protein-Sparing Modified Fast." *Diabetes* 25(1975):494–504.

Boyle, P.C.; Storlien, L.H.; and Keesey, R.E. "Increased Efficiency of Food Utilization Following Weight Loss." *Physiology and Behavior* 21(1978):261–264.

Bray, George A. "Physiological Control of Energy Balance." *International Journal of Obesity* 4(1980):287–295.

Brown, Jerry M. "Cardiac Complication of Protein-Sparing Modified Fasting." *Journal of the American Medical Association* 240(1978):120–122.

Durrant, Merril L.; and Garrow, J.S. "The Effect of Increasing the Relative Cost of Palatable Food with Respect to Ordinary Food on Total Energy Intake of Eight Obese Inpatients." *International Journal of Obesity* 6(1982):153–164.

Dwyer, Johanna T. "Twelve Popular Diets: Brief Nutritional Analyses." *Psychiatric Clinics of North America* 1(1978):621–628.

Faust, Irving M. "Diet-Induced Adipocyte Number Increase in Adult Rats: A New Model of Obesity." *American Journal of Physiology* 235(1978):E279–E286.

Fisler, Janis S. "Nitrogen Economy During Very Low Calorie Reducing Diets: Quality and Quantity of Dietary Protein." *American Journal of Clinical Nutrition* 35(1982):471–486.

Fouty, Robert A. "Liquid Protein Diet, Magnesium Deficiency, and Cardiac Arrest." *Journal of the American Medical Association* 240(1978):2632–2633.

Garn, Stanley M., and Clark, Diane C. "Nutrition, Growth, Development and Maturation: Findings from the Ten-State Nutrition Survey of 1968–1970." *Pediatrics* 56(1975):306–319.

Hegsted, D. Mark. "Dietary Standards." *Journal of the American Dietetic Association* 66(1975):13–21.

Iselin, Hana V., and Burckhardt, Peter. "Balanced Hypocaloric Diet Versus Protein-Sparing Modified Fast in the Treatment of Obesity: A Comparative Study." *International Journal of Obesity* 6(1982):175–181.

Jakubczak, Leonard F. "Calorie and Water Intake as a Function of Strain, Age and Caloric-Density of the Diet." *Physiology and Behavior* 20(1978):273–278.

Khosha, T., and Billewicz, W.Z. "Measurement of Changes in Body Weight." *British Journal of Nutrition* 18(1964):227–239.

Lansky, David, and Brownell, Kelly D. "Estimates of Food Quantity and Calories: Errors in Self-Reporting Among Obese Patients." *American Journal of Clinical Nutrition* 35(1982):727–732.

Miller, Peter M., and Sims, Karen L. "Evaluation and Component Analysis of a Comprehensive Weight Control Program." *International Journal of Obesity* 5(1981):57–65.

Rabast, V.; Schonborn, J.; and Kasper, H. "Dietetic Treatment of Obesity with Low and High-Carbohydrate Diets: Comparative Studies and Clinical Results." *International Journal of Obesity* 3(1979):201–211.

Stunkard, Albert J. "Obesity: Basic Mechanisms Which Regulate Body Weight." *Psychiatric Clinics of North America* 1(1978):459–472.

Van Itallie, Theodore B. "Dietary Approaches to the Treatment of Obesity." *Psychiatric Clinics of North America* 1(1978):609–620.

Van Itallie, Theodore B., and Campbell, Robert G. "Multidisciplinary Approach to the Problem of Obesity." *Journal of the American Dietetic Association* 61(1972):385–390.

Van Itallie, Theodore B., and Yang, Mei Uih. "Current Concepts in Nutrition. Diet and Weight Loss." *New England Journal of Medicine* 297(1977):1158–1161.

Yang, Mei U., and Van Itallie, Theodore B. "Composition of Weight Lost During Short-Term Weight Reduction: Metabolic Responses of Obese Subjects to Starvation and Low-Calorie Ketogenic and Nonketogenic Diets." *Journal of Clinical Investigation* 58(1976):722.

Counseling for Eating Patterns Low in Fat and Cholesterol

Objectives for Chapter 5

1. Identify common dietary misconceptions about fat- and cholesterol-modified patterns that lead to inappropriate eating behaviors.
2. Identify common dietary excesses that contribute to inappropriate eating behaviors associated with diets low in fat and cholesterol.
3. Identify specific nutrients that should be emphasized in assessing a baseline eating pattern before providing dietary instruction.
4. Identify strategies to treat inappropriate behaviors associated with fat- and cholesterol-modified eating patterns.
5. Generate strategies to deal with clients following low-fat and low-cholesterol eating patterns.
6. Identify elements necessary for both client and counselor evaluation.
7. Recommend dietary adherence tools for clients on fat- and cholesterol-modified eating patterns.

5

INAPPROPRIATE EATING BEHAVIORS

Diet instructions modified for fat and cholesterol tend to include a variety of problems associated with false information that can lead to inappropriate eating behaviors.

A common problem many clients face is use of commercial products. Keeping abreast of information on new fat-containing products must be a continuing effort by both nutrition counselors and their clients. Clients could develop and use a shopping guide to determine whether new products are low or high in fat, as in Exhibit 5-1. This information is based on the labels; more specific data can be obtained by writing to the manufacturers.

A frequent problem is the mistaken idea that all vegetable oils are low in saturated fat. A client might exclaim joyously: "This palm oil listed on the label is probably okay on my diet since it is vegetable oil." Unfortunately for such clients, palm oil is highly saturated. Another misconception is that eggs alone cause elevated cholesterol levels. A client might declare: "As long as I cut out eggs in my diet, I don't need to worry." In fact, foods low in cholesterol and high in saturated fat, e.g., palm oil and coconut oil, also elevate serum cholesterol.

Some clients feel that certain foods possess strange powers to cut cholesterol and therefore lower its concentration in the blood. They see single foods as a panacea. A client might claim: "I eat large amounts of fruits and vegetables so I don't worry about my cholesterol intake." The total diet must be considered when assessing fat and cholesterol intake. Single foods do not eliminate the effect of fat and cholesterol in the diet.

Still another erroneous idea is that total fat content does not really matter. As long as a high-fat item is cholesterol free, clients may believe mistakenly that it can be eaten in unlimited quantities. A client might state proudly: "I eat large amounts of peanut butter because it is cholesterol

Exhibit 5–1 Shoppers' Guide to Low Cholesterol

Date: _____

Breads

Acceptable
Sourdough Toast (Wasa)
The following mixes, prepared with home fat:
  Honey French Sourdough Bread Mix (Goldrush)
  Wheatberry Sourdough Bread Mix (Goldrush)
  Bran and Buttermilk Sourdough Bread Mix (Goldrush)
  Sourdough Pancake and Waffle Mix: Whole Wheat, Honey, Buttermilk varieties
  (Goldrush)
  Buttermilk Pancake Mix (Martha White)

Cereals
Acceptable
Back to Nature (Organic Milling Co.)
  Almond Crisp   No added fat
  Raisin Bran Crunch   No added fat
*To be avoided (too high in total fat and
contain saturated fat)*
Golden Harvest (Natural Sales Co.):   Fat (gms/100 gms)
  Apple Bran   24.7—soybean oil, coconut
  Old Fashioned Granola   14.1—soybean oil, coconut
  Premier Granola   21.2—soybean oil, coconut

Sauces, Seasonings, Gravies
Acceptable
Picanto Sauce (Tostitos)   No fat

Snacks
(Relatively high in fat; Use only _____ *)
For use with discretion
  Potato Chips, regular and barbecue   Approx. 40% fat—liquid cottonseed oil
    flavor (Charles Chips)
  Natural Flavor Potato Chips (Health   Approx. 40% fat—safflower oil
    Valley)
  Natural Flavor Bran Corn Chips   Approx. 37% fat—safflower oil

Miscellaneous
To be avoided (Too high in total fat and contain saturated fat)
                                         Fat (gms/100 gms)
  On-Yos Salad Topping (General Mills)   37—partially hydrogenated vegetable oil
                                           (soybean, palm, cottonseed)
  Nut-Os Salad Topping (General Mills)   31—vegetable oil (coconut, cottonseed, sun-
                                           flower seed, peanut, soybean)

*The amount specified will depend on the particular diet prescription for each client.

---

free." This statement is true but large quantities of fat elevate the caloric level of the diet and can lead to weight gain.

These misconceptions are by no means the only ones that clients will voice. They are, however, very common sources of problem eating behaviors. Nutrition counselors cannot follow clients around checking on their daily eating behaviors so, in some cases, they can consume commercial products containing saturated fat without detection for long periods.

Clients following fat- and cholesterol-modified eating patterns must wrestle with problems of excess much like those on weight-control diets. Social pressures can lead clients to eat something they know increases cholesterol, with the familiar alibi: "I just couldn't stop with one bite of that cheesecake at the party last night." These eating patterns also may mean a drastic reduction in the amounts of foods clients are accustomed to eating. They may comment: "No one can live on this small amount of meat."

Inappropriate eating behaviors may be a direct result of childhood excesses. The stalwart farmer may declare: "I grew up eating three eggs every morning."

Manufacturers have jumped to the aid of clients who must follow fat-modified diets by providing either "filled" products or nearly fat-free substitutes. The "filled" products are those that may, for example, have animal fat removed and a polyunsaturated fat added. Others may have all animal fat removed, with no polyunsaturated fat replacement. This can leave the product virtually fat free. Unfortunately, in many cases clients anticipate that these new products will be identical in taste to the originals so frustration and even anger may result when those expectations are not met. In desperation, they may revert to old eating habits, including products high in animal fat.

Clients equate excesses with the prevention of medical problems. In the author's experience, many have used this reasoning: "I use large amounts of oil and margarines extremely high in polyunsaturated fat because I know polyunsaturated fat lowers cholesterol." These inappropriate eating behaviors can lead to excess, unwanted calories. Clients must learn first to examine ways to cut back on saturated fats.

ASSESSMENT OF EATING BEHAVIORS

In assessment of clients who are following fat- and cholesterol-modified eating patterns, the approach should not be one of trying to determine one problem from among a myriad of psychological, social, and behavioral difficulties. Rather, the main problem is known: they must follow a diet to help lower their serum cholesterol levels. Their motivation is one of health, usually unclouded by personal appearance, such as with weight control. In this type of case, the clients may be inexperienced in dealing with eating changes so the counselors' approach will be much different from that in dealing with individuals who have tried to lose weight and failed.

In this type of situation, the counselors' first task is to collect data to use in formulating a dietary pattern tailored to each client. Each pattern should be adjusted to meet a specific dietary prescription that is appropriate for each client.

Assessment in cases involving fat-modified diets can be more specific than in weight-loss regimens. Four crucial components of the diet should be assessed: (1) cholesterol, (2) saturated fat, (3) polyunsaturated fat, and (4) total dietary fat.

During assessment, the list of foods used to complete a quantified food frequency chart might include the foods listed in Exhibit 5–2. This list can be increased or abbreviated depending upon the information needed in formulating a dietary pattern. A seven-day diet record should be used to supplement this information. These data will include amounts of cholesterol, saturated, polyunsaturated, and total fats and information on inappropriate regular eating patterns.

The review of the dietary data should indicate where a major problem is occurring—cholesterol content, saturated fat content, or both. Identification of where the major excess lies will lead to a plan for dietary change focused on strategies to help eliminate the inappropriate patterns.

TREATMENT STRATEGIES

With a clear description of the problem, counselors can begin tailoring the diet to specific client needs. Tailoring involves more than just adapting a standard fat-modified diet instruction sheet; a major element is calculating a pattern compatible with the prescription and the clients' previous daily eating behavior.

A hypothetical example of how tailoring might work in one individual's situation follows.

Mrs. S. eats seven eggs each week and six ounces of meat a day, drinks only skim milk, and uses four teaspoons of margarine (soft, tub, nondiet) with two teaspoons of Mazola oil. She loves eggs and has eaten only high-fat meats such as bologna, salami, beef wieners, etc. Based on her blood values and past health history, the dietary prescription agreed upon by the medical team is 200 milligrams of cholesterol, P/S ratio (polyunsaturated fat divided by saturated fat) of 1.0, and total fat 20–25 percent of total calories.

Exhibit 5–2 Fat and Cholesterol Intake Monitor

Name _____ Visit No. _____ Date _____

	Amount	Chol. (mg.)	Total Fat (gm.)	Sat. Fat (gm.)	Poly. Fat (gm.)	Minimum Significant Amount
Eggs						½ mo
Bacon						4 strips/mo
Sausage						2 oz/mo
Meat Lunch						
Dinner						
Luncheon Meat						See sausage
Shrimp						2 oz/mo
Pork, Beef						3 oz/6 mo
Liver, Chicken						1 oz/2 mo
Gravy						1 cup/mo
Milk, whole___						½ cup/wk
2%___						1 cup/wk
Cheese ___						1 oz/2 wks
Cottage Cheese						½ cup/2 wks
Cream—Light, Sour						1 tb/wk
Heavy						1 tb/mo
Half and Half						1 tb/wk
Nondairy						1 tb/wk
Creamer						
Ice Cream						½ cup/mo
Ice Milk						1 cup/mo
Butter						1 tsp/2 wks
Margarine (as spread)						
_____						1 tsp/wk
(in cooking)						
_____						1 tsp/wk
Salad Dressing						
_____						1 tb/wk
*Breaded Fried Foods						
_____						1 tsp/wk
*Fried Potatoes						
_____						1 tsp/wk
*Baked Products						
_____						1 sv/mo
*Snack Foods						
Chocolate						½ oz/wk
Peanut Butter						1 tb/wk
Nuts						4 tb/mo
Total						

Polyunsaturated fat ÷ saturated fat (P/S) = _____

Exhibit 5–2 continued

*For use in calculating:	Yields		Yields
3–4″ diameter pancakes	1 tsp. fat	15 pieces of French fried	
1 fried egg	1 tsp. fat	potatoes (½″x½″x½″)	2 tsp. fat
1 tbsp. of salad dressing	1½ tsp. fat	½ cup pan fried potatoes	2 tsp. fat
1 oz. pan fried meat, fish		cake with frosting	
and poultry	½ tsp. fat	(1 piece, 2″x3″x2″)	3 tsp. fat
1 oz. breaded and fried meat,		pie (1 piece, 1/7th of 9″)	4 tsp. fat
fish and poultry	1 tsp. fat	cookies (4 pieces, 3″ diam.)	3 tsp. fat
		doughnuts and sweet rolls	
		(1 piece, 4″ diam.)	2 tsp. fat
		crackers and chips (excluding	
		low-fat crackers) (12 pieces)	3 tsp. fat

Source: Joan Bickel, Karen Smith, Linda G. Snetselaar, and Laura Vailas.

Table 5–1 Example of a Tailoring Pattern

	Cholesterol*	Total Fat**	Saturated Fat†	Polyun- saturated Fat†	
3 eggs/week	108	2.5	.73	.30	
4 oz. meat/day	108	14.0	5.48	1.08	
0 dairy (fat)	—	—	—	—	
3 teaspoons Fleischmann's tub margarine/day		11.1	2.10	4.71	
2 teaspoons Mazola oil/day	—	9.4	1.24	5.66	P/S
Total	216	37.0	9.55	11.75	1.23
(% of 1500 calories)		(22%)		(7%)	

* *Figures are calculated to the nearest whole number.*
** *Figures are calculated to the nearest tenth.*
† *Figures are calculated to the nearest hundredth.*

Table 5–1 offers a possible dietary pattern designed to incorporate this basic information and still meet the prescription.

This is an example of how to set a regimen designed to give success initially because it is tailored to past eating habits. Clients should be cautioned that there always will be compromises and that changes will be necessary to meet a specific prescription.

The clients should tailor other elements of the diet while working it into their life style. For example, an alteration in Mrs. S.'s diet may involve eliminating some of the seven eggs she eats each week. She may need to experiment with low-fat breakfast items such as cereal, English muffins, etc.

Once clients and counselors agree on the pattern, instruction on the diet can begin. This consists of planned steps beginning with tasks accomplished most easily, then working up to the more difficult ones. This is called staging the diet instruction.

For example, Mrs. S. is not a dairy product lover and eats high-fat dairy products only occasionally. Her program would begin by working to eliminate all such products and on arranging substitutes. The next step would be changing the amounts and types of meats eaten. Finally, eggs are her "first love" and it will be difficult to eliminate them or to work in alternate foods.

Each of these three changes can be accomplished gradually during separate interviews or telephone conversations. Either way, time should be allowed for the clients to try out ideas in daily life before moving on to more difficult changes.

In addition to dietary changes, misconceptions should be addressed. A few of those were covered earlier in this chapter. Others include comments that:

- "All pork is forbidden on low-cholesterol diets." In reality, lean pork is lower in saturated fat than is beef.
- "If I fry commercial pork sausage until it's brown, all of the fat is removed." It is impossible to remove all fat from high-fat meats such as pork sausage.
- "I use a lot of nondairy powdered whipped toppings because they contain coconut oil rather than dairy fat." Coconut oil is a highly saturated vegetable oil so clients should avoid consuming it in large quantities.

To help clear up misconceptions, counselors should provide a list of commercial and noncommercial foods such as that in Exhibit 5–1 (supra).

Counselors also should build a resource file of manufactured food products through letters like that in Exhibit 5–3. The letters should be concise and to the point. They should be specific as to the types of information requested; in this case, the only interest is fat content. In some instances, additional information on, for example, carbohydrates, protein, etc., can be requested.

While information on manufactured products is valuable, clients also will need to know how to alter old eating habits on social occasions. In

Exhibit 5–3 First Step in Building a Resource File

August 11, 1983

Bonnell Soup Company
1000 East Main Street
Anytown, U.S. 99999

Dear Sirs:

Since we are involved in counseling many hundreds of patients on cholesterol and fat-controlled diets, we often need the assistance of food manufacturers. Determining the exact composition of products allows us to incorporate them into diets, where otherwise they might be prohibited.

Would you please send us your latest figures on the levels of cholesterol, monounsaturated, polyunsaturated, and saturated fatty acids in your Italian Spaghetti with Meatballs. Figures on a per weight basis are most useful to us.

We would appreciate this information at your earliest possible convenience. Thank you for your help and cooperation.

Sincerely yours,

John Smith, R.D., M.S.
Research Nutritionist

the past, food was considered a symbol of gratitude, love, and celebration on special occasions—associations that can make changing old eating habits at such events very unpleasant or difficult.

Changes in eating behavior can be made easier if clients can make clear to helping friends and relatives why the new pattern is necessary. For example, clients can explain that cutting down on cholesterol and saturated fats can help in treating possible heart problems. Such a rationale can encourage these helping others who are hosting the parties to serve foods that are low in cholesterol and saturated fat.

On their own, clients will find that a positive step is to learn to avoid foods that are high in fat and/or cholesterol and to limit their intake to those that are lower in these elements. Figure 5–1 shows a food list that allows for holiday treats.

Figure 5–1 Watch the Lights for Eating at Parties

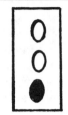 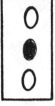 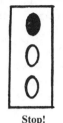

Go Ahead!		**Proceed Slowly!**	**Stop!**
Finger Foods		*Meat Appetizers*	Chicken livers
Carrot sticks	Tomatoes	Shrimp	
Celery sticks	Mush-	Crab	Hors d'oeuvres wrapped in
Cauliflower	rooms	Chicken and ham salad	bacon
Radishes	Pickles	Sweet and sour pork	Cocktail wieners and
Lettuce	Arti-	Fish	sausages
Cabbage	chokes		Braunschweiger
	Avocado	*Party Munchies*	Chopped liver, liver
Sauces and		Potato chips	pâté
Spreads	*Fruits*	Cheese nibbles	
Cocktail sauce	All kinds:	Corn chips	Cheese and chocolate
Sweet and sours	Fresh	Party crackers	fondues (unless you can
Peanut butter	Frozen		stop at one bite)
	Canned	*Dips and Nibbles*	
Low-Fat		(Use only skim milk	Chocolate candies
Munchies		the rest of the day)	
Pretzels	Oyster	Low-fat yogurt dips	Commercial snacks
Rye crisps	crackers		containing high-fat crust
Saltines	Graham	*Pizza Hors D'Oeuvres*	(eggrolls, tarts, etc.)
Popcorn, no	crackers		
butter	Melba toast	*Fruit Breads and Cakes*	Cream cheese appetizers
Bread, white,	Bread sticks		
rye and			Sour cream dips
pumpernickel	*Nuts*		
	Peanuts		
Candy	Pecans		
Gumdrops	Brazil nuts		
Hard candies	Almonds		
Peanut brittle	Cashews		
Beverages			
Soft drinks			
Fruit punches			
Alcoholic			
beverages			
(without egg			
or cream)			

Source: Karen Smith and Linda G. Snetselaar.

Families can do much to help clients in adhering to a fat-modified diet. Nutrition counselors should involve family members in sessions in which the clients are taught food preparation and receive dietary recommendations. However, too much family involvement can pose problems.

For example, a quiet hyperlipidemic teenager may have a mother who volunteers all information and allows no verbal contact between client and counselor. The counselor may decide to see the client alone for parts of the interview or use subtle extinction techniques and nonverbal (i.e., no eye contact) gestures to curb too much involvement by the mother. The counselor might state at the beginning of the interview, "Mrs. J., during today's session I would like to find out from your son what his eating habits are at school. When he has finished, I will ask you to help him in describing eating habits at home." It is important to keep good eye contact with the son to encourage his responses rather than his mother's.

Counselors should instruct the clients' friends and other family members (if possible) on how to provide positive reinforcement as a way to improve the individuals' adherence to a fat-modified diet. The following is a checklist family members might use for positive reinforcement techniques. They should:

- Praise efforts at decreasing serving sizes of meat, cheese, eggs, and other high-fat, high-cholesterol products.
- Avoid teasing or tempting with high-fat, high-cholesterol foods.
- Record the number of positive and negative comments they make about the diet and try to increase the positive and decrease the negative ones.
- Avoid referring to low-cholesterol fat-modified foods as "different" or "strange."

Good basic nutrition should play a primary role in devising a fat-modified diet pattern. The Food and Nutrition Board has not established a Recommended Dietary Allowance for fat.[1] It does recommend that adequate lipids be incorporated into the diet to provide the body with essential fatty acids and carriers of fat-soluable vitamins. Ingesting 15 to 25 grams of fat per day normally will meet this requirement.

Studies in both humans and animals have shown that the necessary requirement for essential fatty acids is fulfilled when 1 to 2 percent of the total caloric intake is provided by linoleic acid.[2,3] A diet of 1,500 calories should provide 1.5 to 3.0 grams of linoleic acid. This is accomplished easily by using vegetable oils in cooking and salad dressing. Corn, soy, and cottonseed oils each contain 6 to 8 grams of linoleic acid per tablespoon, mayonnaise 6 grams, and margarines from 1 to 5 grams.

The United Nations Committee on Dietary Allowances also places a ceiling on the amount of polyunsaturated fat consumed in a day. The committee recommends not exceeding 10 percent of dietary calories as polyunsaturated fat.[4,5] The counselors should begin decreasing saturated fat in clients' diets, thereby automatically increasing the P/S ratio of the diet. A diet modifying fat and cholesterol should not be started by increasing polyunsaturated fat without first decreasing saturated fat.

EVALUATION OF BEHAVIORS

The next step is evaluating the clients' progress. Food records and/or diet histories may provide needed information to assess adherence to the regimen. Family members can be asked to help in monitoring progress by indicating whether a day's adherence has been excellent, poor, or fair. It is important that the clients agree to this type of monitoring.

The following is a checklist designed to help clients in evaluating their progress:

_____ 1. My dietary patterns have changed but are still compatible with my life style.

_____ 2. My misconceptions about low-cholesterol diets have been replaced with factual information.

_____ 3. Social occasions are less of a problem now than when I first began my diet.

_____ 4. My family provides needed positive reinforcement.

Counselors once again must evaluate their own performance. They might use the following checklist:

_____ 1. Was the assessment before designing the fat- and cholesterol-modified eating pattern adequate to prepare a dietary regimen compatible with the client's life style?

_____ 2. Was the new pattern itself compatible with the client's life style?

_____ 3. Were the strategies to promote dietary adherence to the eating pattern carried out efficiently?

_____ 4. Did I use appropriate verbal and nonverbal interviewing skills in instances where the client might have become disgruntled over my changes in his or her former eating habits?

____ 5. Where might changes have been made?

_____

_____

_____

_____

____ 6. Did I use appropriate counseling skills where dietary adherence to the modified eating pattern was a problem?

____ 7. Where might changes have been made?

_____

_____

_____

_____

____ 8. What general changes would I make in the next counseling interview with a similar client on a fat-modified diet?

_____

_____

_____

_____

Additional checklist items can be supplied for both clients and counselors. Each list should be made more specific as the situations require. The counselor checklist also can be adapted depending on what happened during the interview.

Review of Chapter 5
(Answers in Appendix I)

1. List six dietary misconceptions and excesses related to fat-modified diets that lead to inappropriate eating behaviors.

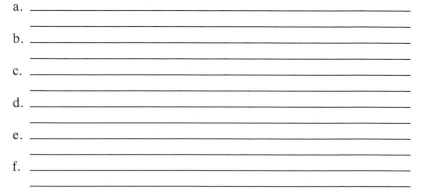

   a. _____

   _____

   b. _____

   _____

   c. _____

   _____

   d. _____

   _____

   e. _____

   _____

   f. _____

   _____

Adherence Tool 5–1 Monitoring Device

Client Meal Planning Chart			
Meal planning can help you in keeping your fat and cholesterol intake low. Before your next visit, plan three days of meals in which you have avoided foods high in fat and cholesterol.			
	Day 1	*Day 2*	*Day 3*
Breakfast:			
Snack:			
Lunch:			
Snack:			
Dinner:			
Snack:			

2. List three specific dietary components of a baseline diet that must be assessed before instructing a client on a fat-modified diet.

   a. _____
   _____

   b. _____
   _____

Adherence Tool 5–2 Informational Device

Tips for Dining in Restaurants

Select from the following suggestions:

Appetizers

Clear soup (bouillon, fat-free consomme). Fruits or vegetables, juices, seafood cocktail (except shrimp), oysters, or clams on the half-shell. (Be sure to count the seafood as part of your meat allowance).

Salads

Lettuce and other vegetables, fruits, fruit and cottage cheese (use as part of milk allowance), gelatin. Use lemon juice, vinegar, vinegar and oil, French dressing, or mayonnaise as your dressing.

Entree

Baked, broiled, or roasted fish, poultry, lean meat, cottage cheese.

Vegetables

All vegetables prepared without butter, meat fat, or cream sauce.

Potatoes and Substitutes

Baked or broiled without dressing, mashed if made without butter, plain rice, macaroni, or spaghetti.

Desserts

Fresh or canned fruits, fruit compotes, sherbert, gelatin, unfrosted angel food cake.

Beverages

Coffee or tea (without cream), carbonated beverages, fruit juices, milk (as allowed), and alcoholic beverages (unless not allowed because of medical problems).

Breakfast Cereals

All cereals without coconut, served with allowed milk.

Miscellaneous

Nuts (except walnuts and filberts), honey, jam, syrup, hard candy, marshmallows, gumdrops, hard fruit drops, jellybeans, mints (no chocolate or bon bons), condiments, and seasoning, as allowed.

Avoid

Combination dishes, fried or creamed foods, foods made with whole milk products, butter, cheese, or gravy. Do not eat pastries (sweet rolls, pies, cakes, cookies, doughnuts, waffles), fatty meats (bacon, sausage, luncheon meats), cream soups, or potato or corn chips.

Inquire about the fat and other ingredients used in menu items. Then give specific instructions regarding the methods of preparation of your selection.

---

c. _____
   _____

3. List three strategies that might help the client follow a fat- and cholesterol-controlled eating pattern:

   a. _____
      _____

   b. _____
      _____

c. _____
_____

4. The following is an exercise (based on Exhibit 5-2) to help you apply the ideas just discussed:

> Jim is a 48-year-old mailman who eats all meals at home except for social occasions, in which he participates frequently. He loves meat and rarely eats eggs or dairy products. Tailor an eating pattern to his needs and explain two counseling strategies that might be used to help his dietary adherence on social occasions. The dietary prescription is 200 milligrams of cholesterol with a P/S ratio of 1.0 and 20 percent of the calories coming from fat.

	Cholesterol	Total Fat	Saturated Fat	Polyun-saturated Fat
__ eggs/week	—	—	—	—
__ ounces meat/day	—	—	—	—
__ ounces whole milk/day	—	—	—	—
__ _____ margarine/day	—	—	—	—
__ _____ oil/day	—	—	—	__ P/S
Total	—	—	—	__ __
(% of 2,400 calories)		(__%)		(__%)

Strategies:_____
_____
_____
_____
_____

5. Identify four possible questions to raise in evaluating client progress:

a. _____
_____

b. _____
_____

c. _____
_____

d. _____
_____

6. Identify six possible questions to review in evaluating your interviewing and counseling skills following a session with a client:

   a. _____

   b. _____

   c. _____

   d. _____

   e. _____

   f. _____

NOTES

1. Food and Nutrition Board, *Recommended Dietary Allowances, 9th ed.*, (Washington, D.C.: National Academy of Sciences, National Research Council, 1980), 33.

2. A.E. Hansen, et al. "Role of Linoleic Acid in Infant Feeding: Clinical and Chemical Study of 428 Infants Fed on Milk Mixtures Varying in Kind and Amount of Fat," *Pediatrics* 31(1963): Supplement.

3. R.T. Holman, W.O. Caster, and H.F. Wiese, "The Essential Fatty Acid Requirement of Infants and the Assessment of Their Dietary Intake of Linoleic by Serum Fatty Acid Analysis," *American Journal of Clinical Nutrition* 14(1964):70.

4. Food and Nutrition Board, *Recommended Allowances*, p. 36.

5. FAO Expert Committee, *Dietary Fats and Oils in Human Nutrition*, FAO Food and Nutrition Paper No. 3. (Rome: United Nations Food and Agriculture Organization.)

SUGGESTED READINGS

Books

American Dietetic Association. *Handbook of Clinical Dietetics*. New Haven, Conn.: Yale University Press, 1981.

Connor, William E., and Connor, Sonja L. *The Alternative Diet Book*. Iowa City, Iowa: University of Iowa, 1976.

Frederickson, Donald S. *Dietary Management of Hyperlipoproteinemia: A Handbook for Physicians and Dietitians*. (U.S. Department of Health, Education, and Welfare, National Institutes of Health, Publication No. [NIH] 75–110). Bethesda, Md.: National Heart, Lung, and Blood Institute, 1974.

Jones, Jeanne. *Diet for a Happy Heart*. San Francisco: 101 Productions, 1975.

Levy, Robert I. *Nutrition in Health and Disease, Vol. I: Nutrition, Lipids and Coronary Heart Disease, A Global View*. New York: Raven Press, 1979.

Rifkind, Basil M., and Levy, Robert I., eds. *Hyperlipidemia, Diagnosis and Therapy*. New York: Grune & Stratton, 1977.

Articles

Anderson, Barbara A.; Fristrom, Geraldine A.; and Weihrauch, John L. "X. Lamb and Veal, Comprehensive Evaluation of Fatty Acids in Foods." *Journal of the American Dietetic Association* 70(1977):53-58.

Anderson, Barbara A.; Kinsella, John A.; and Watt, Bernice K. "II. Beef Products, Comprehensive Evaluation of Fatty Acids in Foods." *Journal of the American Dietetic Association* 67(1975):35-41.

Anderson, Barbara A. "VII. Pork Products, Comprehensive Evaluation of Fatty Acids in Foods." *Journal of the American Dietetic Association* 69(1976):44-49.

Brown, Helen B. "Food Patterns That Lower Blood Lipids in Man." *Journal of the American Dietetic Association* 58(1971):303-311.

Christakis, George; Rinzler, Seymour H.; and Archer, Morton. "Effects of the Anticoronary Club Program on Coronary Heart Disease Risk-Factor Status." *Journal of the American Medical Association* 198(1966):597-604.

Connor, William L., and Connor, Sonja L. "The Key Role of Nutritional Factors in the Prevention of Heart Disease." *Preventive Medicine,* 1(1972):49-83.

Connor, William. "The Effects of Dietary Carbohydrate on the Serum Lipids in Human Subjects." *Circulation* (Supplement III) 40(1969):III-61.

Fristrom, Geraldine A., and Weihrauch, John L. "VIII. Fowl, Comprehensive Evaluation of Fatty Acids in Foods." *Journal of the American Dietetic Association* 69(1976):517-522.

Glueck, Charles L., and Connor, William E. "Diet-Coronary Heart Disease Relationships Reconnoitered." *American Journal of Clinical Nutrition* 31(1978):727-737.

Grande, Francisco; Anderson, Joseph T.; and Keys, Ancel. "Diets of Different Fatty Acid Composition Producing Identical Serum Cholesterol Levels in Man." *American Journal of Clinical Nutrition* 25(1972):53-60.

Hall, Yolanda. "Effectiveness of a Low Saturated Fat, Low Cholesterol, Weight Reducing Diet for the Control of Hypertriglyceridemia." *Atherosclerosis* 16(1972):389-403.

Heysted, D.M. "Quantitative Effects of Dietary Fat on Serum Cholesterol in Man." *American Journal of Clinical Nutrition* 17(1965):281-295.

Hill, P., and Wynder, E.L. "Dietary Regulation of Serum Lipids in Healthy, Young Adults." *Journal of the American Dietetic Association* 68(1976):25-30.

Lees, Robert S., and Wilson, Dana E. "The Treatment of Hyperlipoproteinemia." *New England Journal of Medicine* 284(1971):186-195.

Levy, Robert I. "Dietary and Drug Treatment of Hyperlipoproteinemia." *Annals of Internal Medicine* 77(1972):267-294.

McMurry, Martha P.; Connor, William E.; and Cerqueira, Maria T. "Dietary Cholesterol and the Plasma Lipids and Lipoproteins in the Tarahumara Indians: A People Habituated to a Low Cholesterol Diet After Weaning." *American Journal of Clinical Nutrition* 35(1982):741-744.

Posati, Linda P.; Kinsella, John E.; and Watt, Bernice K. "I. Dairy Products, Comprehensive Evaluation of Fatty Acids in Foods." *Journal of the American Dietetic Association* 66(1975):482-488.

————. "III. Eggs and Egg Products, Comprehensive Evaluation of Fatty Acids in Foods." *Journal of the American Dietetic Association* 67(1975):111-115.

Wilson, Stan W. "Serial Lipid and Lipoprotein Responses to the American Heart Association Fat-Controlled Diet." *American Journal of Medicine* 51(1971):491-503.

Counseling for Low-Carbohydrate Eating Patterns

Objectives for Chapter 6

1. Identify factors that contribute to common inappropriate behaviors associated with carbohydrate-modified eating patterns.
2. Identify specific nutrients that should be emphasized in assessing a baseline eating pattern   before providing dietary instruction.
3. Identify strategies to help combat inappropriate eating behaviors.
4. Generate strategies to deal with clients following carbohydrate-modified eating patterns.
5. Identify elements necessary for both client and counselor evaluation.
6. Recommend dietary adherence tools for clients on carbohydrate-modified eating patterns.

6

INAPPROPRIATE EATING BEHAVIORS

Carbohydrate-modified regimens can include diets such as the diabetic, simple sugar restricted, restricted carbohydrate (increased protein and fat), lactose restricted, and a variety of other less frequently used restrictions. Carbohydrate modifications are approached here in a very general manner, with emphasis on the diabetic diet. Many of the problems with this type of eating pattern are similar to those seen in other types of altered eating patterns.

Any survey of the problems associated with carbohydrate-modified eating patterns makes clear that much of today's social eating activities revolve around carbohydrates: the birthday, wedding, and anniversary cakes; the party mints; the boxes of chocolates; the holiday cookies and candies . . . the list is endless.

Because social pressures may dictate what is eaten on special occasions, nutrition counselors frequently will hear clients' statements such as: "But it's my birthday!"

Carbohydrates also have been associated frequently with emotions such as love, gratitude, mutual feelings of joy, etc. When dietary modification is approached, the association of foods and these deep emotions leads to changes in old eating habits that can be achieved only with the greatest difficulty. Nutrition counselors will hear comments such as: "But I have a sweet tooth," or "Everything I love contains carbohydrates."

The food industry has tried to provide substitutes for the old stand-by sugar. Many clients will respond: "You expect me to eat those brownies made with sugar substitutes? They have a very strange aftertaste."

ASSESSMENT OF EATING BEHAVIORS

Nutrition counselors should use three essential components to facilitate problem solving during interviews:

1. assessment
2. treatment
3. evaluation.

A careful assessment of individual eating behaviors before instructing clients on a carbohydrate-modified eating pattern is essential. Too often the first step is the instruction, not the assessment.

Counselors should begin by collecting data on the simple and complex carbohydrate content of the diet. By asking clients to provide a record of intake over a period of three to seven days, counselors involve these individuals in the process of changing their eating behaviors. The clients begin to feel as though control can be self-regulated, with the counselors becoming facilitators.

Once the baseline carbohydrate content is identified, the general problems the clients will face in following the diet become obvious. Counselors should work with clients in making a list of these problems. For the purpose of problem identification, the use of food items identified as high or low in complex or simple sugars can be more practical than using the exact carbohydrate figures in grams.

Clients should help in identifying the major area that should be the first target in making a carbohydrate modification. That area should be used as a main topic for the next in-depth interview. This provides structure and allows concentration of efforts on one specific behavior. It is obvious, of course, that with a diabetic, the entire diet must be followed from the beginning in order to provide optimum insulin regulation. However, as problems in adhering to the regimen arise, solutions can be staged and worked on gradually.

TREATMENT STRATEGIES

The next step is to determine inappropriate eating patterns that are initiated by specific circumstances and followed by specific consequences— what activity or thought precedes and follows an eating behavior—and developing ways of coping with (or treating) the situations. For example, a teenager has a problem eliminating a midafternoon candy bar and substituting fresh fruit. By identifying the activity or thoughts before the candy bar is eaten, nutritionists can help the youth reprogram thoughts or activities to allow for eating an apple instead:

> CLIENT: "At 3 in the afternoon I always walk by the vending machine. Those candy bars are so tempting I tell myself I deserve a reward for studying so hard all day and I take one. Then I feel terrible, mentally, after eating it."
>
> NUTRITION COUNSELOR: "What would happen if you brought an apple from home and placed it in your locker?"
>
> CLIENT: "Sure, then I could walk past the locker, get the apple, and eat it instead of the candy. I could bypass the vending machines."
>
> NUTRITION COUNSELOR: "It would be all right to pat yourself on the back a bit and say, 'I really feel good. I'm not hungry and ate a food that's good for me!' "

Another strategy is tailoring, which relies heavily on the information collected during dietary assessment. Tailoring for the diabetic is very important because it will help increase adherence to the regimen. An example of tailoring a modified eating pattern is:

> CLIENT: "I really miss drinking orange juice at breakfast. But according to this standard pattern, I can't have it in addition to a fresh fruit that I also like."
>
> NUTRITION COUNSELOR: "We can work out a sample menu using a smaller portion of the fresh fruit so you still can drink a small glass of orange juice."

Tailoring a carbohydrate-modified diet also may mean working with sugar substitutes and determining whether they will be acceptable to the clients. For some clients a reward may be inclusion of desserts that might have been forbidden otherwise. Others will refuse to use sugar substitutes and it may be necessary to reach a compromise in which fresh or water-packed fruits are used as desserts instead of the favorite high-carbohydrate foods. To improve self-thoughts, clients can record positive and negative monologues, then try to increase the positive ones involving appropriate eating behaviors. (The Appendix F form can be used.)

With a diabetic diet, which distributes carbohydrates in set amounts throughout the day, the pattern takes on a more rigid nature. There is less flexibility in shifting nutrients from one meal to another. The last example demonstrates that additional rigidity but still permits some compromise.

Staging the diet is very important. This is accomplished by concentrating on one problem at a time. It involves a gradual, procedural approach to maintaining adherence.

Staging plays a large role in helping to target certain problem areas:

> CLIENT: "I see that I'm really going to have problems following this diet in the morning, particularly during my 10 o'clock break."
>
> NUTRITION COUNSELOR: "Okay, we will concentrate on this problem. At the next visit we will discuss how your attempts to alleviate it worked."

Because consumption of high-carbohydrate foods is a substantial part of most people's social lives, changing dietary habits to restrict or eliminate them can pose problems. In analyzing social occasions, nutrition counselors should always try to identify antecedents and consequences (events or thoughts preceding and following eating behaviors). This in essence identifies conduct that prompts certain eating patterns. In social situations this is very important:

> CLIENT: "I really have problems controlling my carbohydrate intake while I'm at parties."
>
> NUTRITION COUNSELOR: "Describe for me an actual situation during a party in which you had this difficulty."
>
> CLIENT: "My friend, Marge, had thrown a birthday party for me. While I was talking with some friends she walked over to me and said, 'Please take some of these chocolates. I slaved all day making them for you.' "
>
> NUTRITION COUNSELOR: "What was your response?"
>
> CLIENT: "Well, what could I do but just take one and thank her?"
>
> NUTRITION COUNSELOR: "What were you thinking before you took one?"
>
> CLIENT: "I was thinking, 'How can I say 'No' in front of all my friends? Marge went to so much trouble. I can't go into a long explanation about my diet now.' "
>
> NUTRITION COUNSELOR: "What were your thoughts after eating the candy?"
>
> CLIENT: "I thought, 'How could you do such a thing? You know you shouldn't eat that.' "
>
> NUTRITION COUNSELOR: "Let's go back to the beginning. What else could you have done when Marge offered you the candy?"
>
> CLIENT: "Well, I could have thanked her and just explained briefly about my new diet."

NUTRITION COUNSELOR: "Great idea. You also could have mentioned other foods Marge had made and pointed out that you were allowed to eat them. You also might have complimented her on how delicious those were."

CLIENT: "Yes, I think I also would have felt better afterward if things had happened that way."

NUTRITION COUNSELOR: That would be a good time to use some positive self-thought. For example, 'I handled that situation really well.' "

Many clients are part of a family so their problems involve that group as well in many cases. Attempts should be made to include the family in at least part of all phases of nutrition counseling. The family member who prepares the meals should know just as much about the diet as the client.

The family also plays a crucial role in keeping client adherence to the diet stable over time by providing needed positive reinforcement. Counselors should teach each family member to reinforce clients' good eating behaviors positively. The family members also should be asked to avoid tempting the client with food not allowed on the diet. Temptations can be eliminated if the impermissible products are left on the shelves in the grocery store.

A counselor might try to involve the family from the very beginning of the nutrition interview: "Mrs. A., I appreciate your willingness to sit in on these interview sessions with your husband. The two of you will need to work together if the diet is to help his diabetic condition. Your help and support are crucial to his eventual success with the diet."

EVALUATION OF BEHAVIORS

Evaluation of clients' adherence to a carbohydrate-modified eating pattern once again should involve the family. If the clients permit, family members should be asked to describe how well the individuals follow the diet at home. The clients again should fill in a diet record for three to seven days. It also may be of value to ask them to record positive and negative monologues (Appendix F) during social occasions or at any time when conforming to a new eating behavior is a problem.

A knowledge of nutrition is extremely important in work with low-carbohydrate diets. The Food and Nutrition Board has recommended that a minimum of 50 to 100 grams of carbohydrate be eaten in a day.[1] Consuming fewer than 50 grams could result in potentially harmful fat and protein catabolism.[2] Unfortunately, the precise requirement for dietary carbohydrates in humans is not known.

In diabetic clients, the absolute or relative lack of insulin leads to abnormalities in the metabolism of carbohydrates, protein, and fat. Nutrition counselors work with the diabetics to develop a daily diet that contains appropriate amounts of carbohydrate, protein, and fat.[3,4,5]

The American Diabetes Association recommends that 40 percent of an individual's total calories be derived from carbohydrates. Brunzell and coworkers have shown that a higher percent of calories from carbohydrates can be used without compromising the blood glucose levels of insulin-dependent diabetics.[6] The association also recommends that 15 to 20 percent of total calories be derived from protein and 40 to 45 percent from fat. Drash recommends that children receive 55 percent of total calories from carbohydrates (with 65 percent of those from complex carbohydrates), 15 percent of total calories from protein, and 30 percent from fat.[7]

Control of the daily distribution of energy intake is extremely important for diabetics. Skillman and Tzagournis recommend a time of day and fraction of total calories to correspond with labile insulin-requiring stable patients.[8] Scheduling meals at specific times is very important. Skillman and Tzagournis recommend meals at breakfast, noon, supper, and bedtime for stable, insulin-requiring diabetics, with corresponding carbohydrate distributions of 2/7 at breakfast, 2/7 at noon, 2/7 at supper, and 1/7 at bedtime. For labile insulin-requiring diabetics, meals at breakfast, midmorning, noon, afternoon, supper, and bedtime are suggested with carbohydrate distributions of 2/10 at breakfast, 1/10 at midmorning, 2/10 at noon, 1/10 in the afternoon, 3/10 at supper, and 1/10 at bedtime. In noninsulin-requiring stable diabetics, three meals a day are recommended—breakfast, noon, and supper, with the suggested carbohydrate distribution 2/7 at breakfast, 2/7 at noon, and 3/7 at supper. For the noninsulin diabetic caloric intake is also very important.

A checklist for clients to evaluate their eating behaviors might include the following:

_____ 1. Although tailoring the diet to my past habits is difficult, I was able to accomplish it in at least two instances.

_____ 2. My problems with the carbohydrate-modified eating pattern were approached gradually and solved one by one.

_____ 3. I tried to look at eating problems at social occasions by identifying activities or thoughts that preceded or followed consuming an inappropriate food.

_____ 4. My family helps me adhere to the diet by positively reinforcing my good behaviors.

This checklist can be much more exhaustive. Terry provides an excellent method to help evaluate adherence to a diabetic regimen which can supplement the checklist.[9]

Adding specific points in the blanks in the following counselor's checklist could make this instrument more useful for each client:

___ 1. Was the assessment phase of this counseling session adequate to identify potential dietary problems?

___ 2. Did the dietary pattern, although difficult, take into account to the greatest extent possible the client's previous eating behaviors?

___ 3. Did strategies used to promote dietary adherence help the client achieve success in an efficient manner?

___ 4. Did I use appropriate verbal and nonverbal interviewing skills in instances where strategies proved to be ineffective?

___ 5. Where might changes have been made?_____

_____

_____

_____

_____

___ 6. Were the counseling skills used to maintain adherence to the low-carbohydrate eating pattern appropriate?

___ 7. How might changes have been made?_____

_____

_____

_____

_____

_____

___ 8. What general changes would I make in the next counseling interview with a similar client on a carbohydrate-modified diet?

_____

_____

_____

_____

Counselors can revise this checklist so that it will be most useful for their specific needs. If a strategy worked, for example, they might want to record only why they believed it was beneficial. Counselors should be creative with evaluation checklists and should not feel compelled to use pat questions.

As a final step, both client and counselor can develop evaluation checklist items they feel would be most useful for themselves.

Client	Counselor
1. _____	1. _____
2. _____	2. _____
3. _____	3. _____
4. _____	4. _____

Review of Chapter 6
(Answers in Appendix I)

1. List three factors that are commonly associated with carbohydrate-modified diets and lead to inappropriate eating behaviors:
   a. _____
   b. _____
   c. _____
2. List two nutrients to emphasize in collecting baseline information on low-carbohydrate diets.
   a. _____
   b. _____
3. Identify four strategies to help combat inappropriate eating behaviors when working with clients on low-carbohydrate diets:
   a. _____
   b. _____
   c. _____
   d. _____
4. The following describes a problem situation with a client who has been instructed on a diabetic diet. Identify a strategy that might help solve this client's problem and explain your reason for selecting it.

   Mr. J. has been placed on a diabetic diet. During nutrition assessment you found that he has most difficulty with afternoon snacks. At his company during break, everyone eats frosted cup-

Adherence Tool 6–1 Monitoring Device

		No. of Exchanges	Type of Foods and Amount
	One-Day Food Record Name_____		
Breakfast	1. Bread		
	2. Fruit		
	3. Milk		
	4. Meat		
	5. Fat		
Midmorning	1. Bread		
	2. Fruit		
	3. Milk		
	4. Meat		
	5. Fat		
Lunch	1. Bread		
	2. Fruit		
	3. Veg. A		
	4. Veg. B		
	5. Milk		
	6. Meat		
	7. Fat		
Midafternoon	1. Bread		
	2. Fruit		
	3. Milk		
	4. Meat		
	5. Fat		
Dinner	1. Bread		
	2. Fruit		
	3. Veg. A		
	4. Veg. B		
	5. Milk		
	6. Meat		
	7. Fat		
Bedtime	1. Bread		
	2. Fruit		
	3. Milk		
	4. Meat		
	5. Fat		

Adherence Tool 6–2 Informational Device

Menu Planner

Meal 1

_____

_____

_____

_____

_____

Nutrition Guide		
	Rec.*	Act.**
Meat		
Milk		
Fruit & Vegetable		
Bread & Cereal		

Meal 2

_____

_____

_____

_____

_____

_____

Meal 3

_____

_____

_____

_____

_____

_____

Snacks

_____

_____

_____

_____

_____

Source: Nancy L. Schwartz, R.D.   *Rec. = Recommended amounts
**Act. = Actual amounts

cakes, candy bars, or jellybeans. (a) What further questions would you ask to elicit more information? (b) What strategies would you use to help alleviate the problem? (c) Why did you choose these strategies?_____

_____
_____
_____

a. _____
_____
_____
_____

b. _____
_____
_____

c. _____
_____
_____
_____

5. Identify two questions you might evaluate to determine whether or not the client's eating behaviors are changing in the appropriate direction:
   a. _____
   b. _____
6. Identify questions in three general areas you might evaluate to check on how well you as a counselor performed during the counseling session:
   a. _____
   b. _____
   c. _____

NOTES

1. Food and Nutrition Board, *Recommended Dietary Allowances,* 9th ed. (Washington, D.C.: National Academy of Sciences, National Research Council, 1980), 33.

2. D.H. Calloway, "Dietary Components that Yield Energy," *Environmental Biology and Medicine* 1 (1971): 175–186.

3. Robert S. Goodhart and Maurice E. Shils, *Modern Nutrition in Health and Disease* (Philadelphia: Lea and Febiger, 1980), 977–997.

4. Helen S. Mitchell et al., *Nutrition in Health and Disease,* 16th ed. (Philadelphia: J.B. Lippincott Co., 1976), 395–412.

5. Marie V. Krause and L. Kathleen Mahan, *Food, Nutrition and Diet Therapy,* 6th ed. (Philadelphia: W.B. Saunders Company, 1979), 522–542.

6. John D. Brunzell et al., "Effect of a Fat Free, High Carbohydrate Diet on Diabetic Subjects with Fasting Hyperglycemia," *Diabetes* 23 (1974): 138.

7. Allan L. Drash, "Diabetes Mellitus in Childhood: A Review," *Journal of Pediatrics* 78 (1971): 919.

8. T.G. Skillman and M. Tzagournis, *Diabetes Mellitus* (Kalamazoo, Mich.: The Upjohn Company, 1975).

9. Rhonda Dale Terry, "A Model for Comprehensive Diabetes Dietary Care," *The Diabetes Educator* (Fall 1981): 34.

SUGGESTED READINGS

Books

American Diabetes Association and the American Dietetic Association. A Guide for Professionals, The Effective Application of "Exchange Lists for Meal Planning," 1977.

American Dietetic Association. *Handbook of Clinical Dietetics.* New Haven, Conn.: Yale University Press, 1981.

Behrman, D.M. *A Cookbook for Diabetics.* New York: American Diabetes Association, 1959.

Danowski, T.S. *Diabetes As a Way of Life.* 4th rev. ed. New York: Coward, McCann & Geoghegan, 1979.

———, ed. *Diabetes Mellitus, Diagnosis and Treatment.* New York: American Diabetes Association, 1964.

Donahoe, V. *Diabetic Cooking Made Easy.* Minneapolis: Burgess Publishing Company, 1976.

Krall, Leo P. *Joslin Diabetes Manual.* 11th rev. ed. Philadelphia: Lea and Febiger, 1978.

Oakley, Wilfred G.; Pyke, D.A.; and Taylor, W. *Diabetes and Its Management.* 3rd rev. ed. Oxford, England: Blackwell Scientific, 1978.

Revele, Dorothy T. *Gourmet Recipes for Diabetics.* Springfield, Ill.: Charles C Thomas, Publisher, 1971.

Revell, Dorothy. *Oriental Cooking for the Diabetic.* Tokyo: Japan Publications, 1981.

Skillman, T.G., and Tzagournis, M. *Diabetes Mellitus.* Kalamazoo, Mich.: The Upjohn Company, 1975.

Sussman, Karl E., and Metz, Robert J.S., eds. *Diabetes Mellitus.* New York: American Diabetes Association, 1975.

Waiffe, S.O., ed. *Diabetes Mellitus.* 7th rev. ed. Indianapolis: Eli Lilly Company, Lilly Research Laboratories, 1970.

Wolf, Stewart G., and Berle, Beatrice B., eds. *Dilemmas in Diabetes: Advanced Experiments in Medical Biology,* vol. 65. New York: Plenum Press, 1975.

Articles

Albrink, Margaret J. "Dietary and Drug Treatment of Hyperlipidemia in Diabetes." *Diabetes* 23 (1974):913–918.

American Diabetes Association. "Saccharin." *Diabetes Care* 2(1979):380.

Anderson, James W. "Effect of Carbohydrate Restriction and High Carbohydrate Diets on Men with Chemical Diabetes." *American Journal of Clinical Nutrition* 30(1977):402–408.

Anderson, James W. "Metabolic Abnormalities Contributing to Diabetic Complications. I. Glucose Metabolism in Insulin-Insensitive Pathways." *American Journal of Clinical Nutrition* 28(1973):273–280.

Anderson, James W., and Herman, Robert H. "Effects of Carbohydrate Restriction on Glucose Tolerance of Normal Men and Reactive Hypoglycemic Patients." *American Journal of Clinical Nutrition* 28(1975):748–755.

Anderson, James W., and Ward, Kyleen. "Long-Term Effects of High Carbohydrate, High Fiber Diets on Glucose and Lipid Metabolism. A Preliminary Report on Patients with Diabetes." *Diabetes Care* 1(1978):77–82.

Arker, Juanita A.; Gordon, Phillip; and Roth, Jesse. "Defect in Insulin Binding to Receptors in Obese Men: Amelioration with Calorie Restriction." *Journal of Clinical Investigation* 55(1975):166–174.

Arky, Ronald A. "Diet and Diabetes Mellitus." *Postgraduate Medicine* 63(1978):72–78.

Arky, Ronald A.; Wylie-Rosett, J.; and El-Beheri, B. "Examination of Current Dietary Recommendations for Individuals with Diabetes Mellitus." *Diabetes Care* 5(1982):59–63.

Backscheider, Joan F. "Self-Care Requirements, Self-Care Capabilities, and Nursing Systems in the Diabetic Nurse Management Clinic." *American Journal of Public Health* 64(1974):1138–1146.

Bruck, Erika, and MacGillivray, Margaret H. "Posthypoglycemic Hyperglycemia in Diabetic Children." *Journal of Pediatrics* 84(1974):672–680.

Bruhn, John G. "Psychosocial Influences in Diabetes Mellitus." *Postgraduate Medicine* 56(1974):113–118.

Brunzell, John D. "Effects of a Fat Free, High Carbohydrate Diet on Diabetic Subjects with Fasting Hyperglycemia." *Diabetes* 23(1974):138–142.

Brunzell, John D. "Improved Glucose Tolerance with High Carbohydrate Diets with High Carbohydrate Feeding in Mild Diabetes." *New England Journal of Medicine* 284(1971):521–524.

Burgess, Barbara R., and El-Beheri, B. "Rationale for Changes in the Dietary Management of Diabetes." *Journal of the American Diabetic Association* 81(1982):258–261.

Cahill, George F.; Etzwiler, Donnell D.; and Freinkel, Norbert. "Control and Diabetes." *New England Journal of Medicine* 294(1976):1004–1005.

Collier, Greg, and O'Dea, Kerin. "Effects of Physical Form of Carbohydrate on the Postprandial Glucose, Insulin, and Gastric Inhibitory Polypeptide Responses in Type 2 Diabetes." *American Journal of Clinical Nutrition* 36(1982):10–14.

Colwell, John A. "Use of Oral Agents in Treating Diabetes Mellitus." *Postgraduate Medicine* 59(1976):139–144.

Crapo, Phyllis A.; Reaven, Gerald; and Olefsky, Jerrold. "Plasma Glucose and Insulin Responses to Orally Administered Simple and Complex Carbohydrates." *Diabetes* 25(1976):741–747.

Davenport, Rachael R. "Dietitians, Nurses Teach Diabetic Patients." *Hospitals* 48(1974):81–82.

Davidson, John K. "Controlling Diabetes Mellitus with Diet Therapy." *Postgraduate Medicine* 59(1976):114–122.

Doar, J.W.H. "Influence of Treatment with Diet Alone on Oral Glucose-Tolerance Test and Plasma Sugar and Insulin Levels in Patients with Maturity-Onset Diabetes Mellitus." *Lancet* 1(1975):1263–1266.

Drash, Allan L. "Managing the Child with Diabetes Mellitus." *Postgraduate Medicine* 63(1978):85–92.

Dwyer, Lois S., and Fralin, Florence G. "Simplified Meal Planning for Hard to Teach Patients." *American Journal of Nursing* 74(1974):664–665.

Felig, Philip. "Insulin, Glucagon, and Somatostatin in Normal Physiology and Diabetes Mellitus." *Diabetes* 25(1976):1091–1099.

Felig, Phyllis. "Diabetic Ketoacidosis." *New England Journal of Medicine* 290(1974):1360–1363.

Gordon, Edgar S. "Diabetes Mellitus—New Developments." *Postgraduate Medicine* 55(1974):145–149.

Graber, Alan L. "Evaluation of Diabetes Patient-Education Programs." *Diabetes* 26(1977):61–64.

Hinkle, Lawrence E., Jr. "Customs, Emotions, and Behavior in the Dietary Treatment of Diabetes." *Journal of the American Dietetic Association* 41(1962):341–344.

Johnson, Janice B. "Diabetes Education: It Is Not Only What We Say." *Diabetes Care* 5(1982):343–345.

Kaufman, Mildred. "Programmed Instruction Materials on Diabetes." *Journal of the American Dietetic Association* 46(1965):36–38.

Kaufmann, R.L. "Plasma Lipid Levels in Diabetic Children." *Diabetes* 24(1975):672–679.

Kissebah, A.H. "Mode of Insulin Action." *Lancet* 1(1975):144–147.

Kohler, Elaine; Hurwitz, Linda S.; and Milan, Deborah. "A Developmentally Staged Curriculum for Teaching Self-Care to the Child with Insulin-Dependent Diabetes Mellitus." *Diabetes Care* 5(1982):300–304.

Lerner, R.L. "Mechanism of Improved Glucose Tolerance on High Carbohydrate Diets in Normal and Mild Diabetics." *Diabetes* 20(1971):342–343.

MacCuish, A.C. "Antibodies to Pancreatic Islet Cells in Insulin Dependent Diabetics with Coexistent Autoimmune Disease." *Lancet* 2(1974):1529–1531.

Martin, Donald B. "Insulin Resistance: New Insights." *New England Journal of Medicine* 294(1976):778–779.

Maruhama, Yoshisuke. "Dietary Intake and Hyperlipidemia in Controlled Diabetic Outpatients." *Diabetes* 26(1970):94–99.

Maugh, Thomas H. "Diabetes: Epidemiology Suggests a Viral Connection." *Science* 188(1975):347–351.

———. "Diabetes II: Model Systems Indicate Viruses a Cause." *Science* 188(1975):436–438.

McFarlane, Judith, and Hames, Carolyn C. "Children with Diabetes: Learning Self-Care in Camp." *American Journal of Nursing* 73(1973):1362–1365.

Miller, Garifallia. "Diet and Diabetes—New Approach to Planning Meals." *Minnesota Medicine* 55(1972):167–170.

Morrison, Alan S., and Buring, Julie E. "Artificial Sweeteners and Cancer of the Lower Urinary Tract." *New England Journal of Medicine* 302(1980):537–541.

Olefsky, Jerrold M., and Crapo, Phyllis. "Fructose, Xylitol and Sorbitol." *Diabetes Care* 3(1980):390–393.

Owen, Oliver E.; Boden, Guenther; and Shuman, Charles R. "Managing Insulin Dependent Diabetic Patients." *Postgraduate Medicine* 59(1976):127–134.

Partridge, John W. "Attitudes of Adolescents Toward Their Diabetes." *American Journal of Diseases in Children* 124(1972):226–229.

Petrie, J.C.; Stowers, J.M.; and Wood, R.A. "Diabetes Mellitus—Obesity and Dietary Management." *British Medical Journal* 2(1972):706–708.

Power, Lawrence. "New Approaches to the Old Problem of Diabetes Education." *Journal of Nutrition Education* 5(1973):230–232.

Salzar, Joan E. "Classes to Improve Diabetic Self-Care." *American Journal of Nursing* 75(1975):1324–1326.

Schmitt, Barton D. "An Argument for the Unmeasured Diet in Juvenile Diabetes." *Clinical Pediatrics* 14(1975):68–73.

Shagan, Bernard P. "Diabetes in the Elderly Patient." *Medical Clinics of North America* 60(1976):1191–1208.

Stone, Daniel B. "A Rational Approach to Diet and Diabetes." *Journal of the American Dietetic Association* 46(1965):30–35.

Surwit, Richard S.; Scovern, Albert W.; and Feinglos, Mark N. "The Role of Behavior in Diabetes Care." *Diabetes Care* 5(1982):337–342.

Taft, Pincus. "Diet in Management of Diabetics. Why Restrict Carbohydrate?" *The Medical Journal of Australia* 63(1976):838–840.

Tandon, Rakesh K.; Srivastava, L.M.; and Pandey, S.C. "Increased Disaccharidase Activity in Human Diabetics." *American Journal of Clinical Nutrition* 28(1975):621–625.

Tani, Gwens S., and Hankin, Jean H. "A Self-Learning Unit for Patients with Diabetes." *Journal of the American Dietetic Association* 58(1971):331–335.

"University Group Diabetes Study Program: A Study of the Effects of Hypoglycemic Agents and Vascular Complications in Patients with Adult Onset Diabetes." *Diabetes* 19(1970):747–830.

Vinik, A.I.; Kalk, W.J.; and Jackson, W.P.U. "A Unifying Hypothesis for Hereditarily Acquired Diabetes." *Lancet* 1(1974):485–586.

Weinsier, Ronald L. "Diet Therapy of Diabetes—Description of Successful Methodologic Approach to Gaining Diet Adherence." *Diabetes* 23(1974):669–673.

Weinsier, Ronald L. "High and Low Carbohydrate Diets in Diabetes Mellitus." *Annals of Internal Medicine* 80(1974):332–341.

West, Kelly M. "Diet and Diabetes." *Postgraduate Medicine* 60(1976):209–216.

Williams, Franklin T. "The Clinical Picture of Diabetic Control Studied in Four Settings." *American Journal of Public Health* 57(1967):441–451.

Williams, Franklin T. "Dietary Errors Made at Home by Patients with Diabetes." *Journal of the American Dietetic Association* 51(1967):19–25.

Wood, Francis C., and Bierman, Edwin L. "New Concepts in Diabetic Dietetics." *Nutrition Today* 7(1972):4–12.

Wylie-Rosett, Judith. "Development of New Educational Strategies for the Person with Diabetes." *Journal of the American Dietetic Association* 81(1982):268–271.

Other Materials

ADA Forecast (bimonthly) and *ADA Exchange Lists for Meal Planning.* American Diabetes Association, Inc., 1 West 48th Street, New York, N.Y. 10020.

Counseling for Low-Protein Eating Patterns

Objectives for Chapter 7

1. Identify factors that lead to inappropriate eating behaviors associated with protein-modified regimens.
2. Identify specific nutrients that should be emphasized in assessing a baseline eating pattern before providing dietary instruction.
3. Identify strategies to treat inappropriate eating behaviors associated with low-protein patterns.
4. Generate strategies to use in facilitating problem solving for clients who are following a protein-modified eating pattern.
5. Identify elements necessary for both client and counselor evaluation.
6. Recommend dietary adherence tools for clients on protein-modified eating patterns.

7

INAPPROPRIATE EATING BEHAVIORS

Dietary patterns in which protein content is adjusted can take on many forms from one single protein modification to multiple constraints of protein plus potassium, sodium, and fluid. The latter restrictions are associated with a variety of inappropriate eating behaviors.

When instructing clients on a protein, potassium, sodium, and fluid-modified diet, counselors should recall, as noted earlier, that the larger the number of restrictions, the more difficult it will be to follow the diet over time. Clients on this type of diet complain frequently about the changes it requires in their life style. Counselors also should note that the clients are being forced to deal with changes in other areas, such as dialysis. The combination of these factors makes dietary adherence extremely difficult.

As with many other eating patterns, these clients must struggle with social pressures that are multiplied by the large number of restrictions. Clients may drop out of social affairs to avoid the embarrassment of having to explain their health problems.

"Everything in my life has changed!" is a common exclamation. Old eating habits are replaced by a constant preoccupation with restrictions. The tradition of enjoying all food is replaced by a feeling that meals are surrounded by treatment or therapy. For clients with a protein restriction, eating can become only a means toward existence instead of being a "recreational" happening.

New "foreign" foods also are introduced into daily dietary patterns. These substitutes may include low-sodium versions of cheeses, peanut butter, cottage cheese, cornflakes, bread, and crackers. Some nutrition counselors also may recommend low-protein, low-sodium cookies containing aluminum hydroxide, which binds phosphate in the intestines. This medication is necessary for clients with hyperphosphatemia.

173

ASSESSMENT OF EATING BEHAVIORS

Because protein-modified diets can be very difficult to follow, assessment is extremely important.

In its most complicated form, assessment involves identifying the protein content of the diet along with other baseline information as to potassium, sodium, and fluid intake. Using this information as a base, counselors can prepare for tailoring the diet to client needs.

On this basis, counselor and client together can pinpoint where problems may occur, make a list of them, and try to prioritize them. Before ending the assessment session, it is important to identify one general problem that the clients can concentrate on remedying before the next interview.

In addition to the general baseline nutrient level, eating habits should be assessed: times of day, where, and with whom. Where habits conflict with adherence to the diet, possible solutions to such dilemmas should be discussed.

TREATMENT STRATEGIES

A variety of treatment strategies are at the disposal of the nutrition counselors.

One is tailoring. Although many diet restrictions can make tailoring more difficult, it is possible to shape an eating pattern to each individual's likes and dislikes. For example, in the protein category, a variety of meat and meat substitutes are allowed. These should be presented as a means of helping the clients make choices so that the diet will fit in with their life styles and long-term dietary habits.

Counselors should avoid creating the impression that they are the "experts" and in sole control. Too often forms, lists, etc., are presented in a way that leaves the clients feeling totally removed from the whole process of change. They regard themselves as becoming unwilling objects to be moved, shaped, and molded by the counselors. The goal during the sessions should be to include clients in shaping the eating patterns while they continue to follow the dietary prescription.

Staging or prioritizing the components of a diet with several restrictions, all of which must be followed as a package, can be difficult. In this case, staging can take on the solution of one problem area at a time while the clients continue to follow all restrictions to the best of their ability. Once again the clients must be very actively involved in the development of this process. In choosing which problems to tackle first, several factors should be considered:

- Which problem will lead to some success? Initial success can be very important to continued improvement in dietary adherence.
- Which problem is the most difficult and inhibiting from the standpoint of dietary adherence? A very large problem that precludes following the diet may force counselor and client to remedy it first. A client who refuses to comply with any of the dietary recommendations may need first to be attended to by nutritionists or dietitians. Frequently other concerns about the disease lead clients to target one part of their treatment as the reason for dissatisfaction. Attending to clients' feelings may be the first step in solving this problem.
- Which problem is the easiest to solve? That may be a good first choice.

The ultimate choice should be a product of client-counselor teamwork.

Social occasions that call for observance of traditions directly contrary to diet prescriptions can cause adherence problems. To deal with these occasions, identification of events preceding and following a situation involving food can be very valuable in analyzing both the happenings and the clients' thoughts. Both play a great part in changing eating behaviors. For example:

CLIENT: "Everything at the party last night was high in protein."

NUTRITION COUNSELOR: "What did you eat?"

CLIENT: "I just told myself I might as well give up and eat whatever I wanted."

NUTRITION COUNSELOR: "What happened after you ate all of those foods you knew you should not have eaten?"

CLIENT: "I felt terrible mentally. I kept telling myself how rotten I was for not following the diet."

NUTRITION COUNSELOR: "Can you describe for me how you could have handled the situation so you would feel better about the result and about yourself?"

CLIENT: "Well, I suppose I could have tried harder to find foods allowed on my diet. Then I might have felt better about what I was doing."

NUTRITION COUNSELOR: "By feeling better about yourself you begin to give yourself positive reinforcement. That can lead to many excellent eating behaviors."

With many dietary restrictions, alterations in eating style produce problems. A protein-restricted diet may require many commercial substitute foods. Family support in helping clients to learn gradually to use these substitutes can be very important. The counselors should talk with the family about how to gradually add items such as low-sodium peanut butter into the diet. The family should be asked to avoid tempting the client with foods not allowed on the diet or situations where other members comment how unfortunate it is that the individual has to eat a food substitute.

The counselors should encourage the family to get involved with maintaining dietary adherence, particularly by providing techniques for preparing the special (or substitute) foods. In some cases it may be advantageous to allow family members to work on a dietary pattern with the clients. They should be asked to reinforce the clients positively rather than negatively. Examples of ways they can encourage appropriate eating behaviors should be presented: "That's great, you're really doing well with this diet. You know you really have figured out creative ways of using those low-sodium products."

With protein-restricted diets, nutrition again is extremely important. Protein requirements fall into two categories: (1) for essential amino acids, and (2) for the total protein or total nitrogen needed by the body in synthesizing nonessential amino acids and for other nitrogen-containing tissue constituents.

The Recommended Dietary Allowances for essential amino acids vary for different age groups.[1,2] Histidine, isoleucine, leucine, lycine, threonine, tryptophan, and valine are considered essential amino acids. Animal proteins such as meats, poultry, fish, eggs, milk, and cheese provide good quality protein in liberal amounts and are termed complete proteins. Proteins from plant sources are partially complete or incomplete because they lack one or more of the following: lysine, methionine, threonine, and tryptophan. However, these proteins are very important because of their amino acid contribution to the total nitrogen of the body that must be available for nonessential amino acids and other nitrogen-containing compounds in the tissues.

The Food and Nutrition Board also recommends .8 gram of protein per kilogram of body weight for adults. For infants, the recommended allowance is based on the amount of milk protein known to produce a satisfactory growth rate. An additional amount of protein is allowed for growth. In pregnancy, 30 grams per day are added.[3]

Whitney and Hamilton emphasize that the Recommended Dietary Allowances apply to healthy persons only.[4] In clients with renal disease, protein in the diet is increased to 1½ to 2 grams per kilogram of body weight for adults to compensate for urinary losses even though the level of blood urea nitrogen (BUN) is moderately elevated (40 to 60 milligrams per 100 milliliters).[5] For children with renal disease the protein in the diet also would be increased. High biological value proteins should be used to supply 60 to 70 percent of total protein in the diet pattern.[6] High biological value proteins carry most of their nitrogen in their essential amino acids and contain all essential amino acids.

In end-stage renal failure, nitrogen is retained. Blood urea nitrogen is more than 100 milligrams per 100 milliliters. In such a case, the protein in the diet is restricted.[7] At that time the protein needs of the body must be met by proteins of high biological value. The foods that best supply protein in this situation are milk and eggs. Meats also satisfy the criteria but contain somewhat more nitrogen from nonessential amino acids than do milk and eggs.

Clients following a renal diet may need to increase or decrease sodium and potassium, depending on the stage of the disease. Modification in phosphate and vitamin and mineral balance may be required. Each of these problems requires a tremendous effort by nutrition counselors because clients, with so many dietary adjustments to make, need a great deal of advice on how to facilitate change and make the new mode habitual.

EVALUATION OF BEHAVIORS

Particularly with clients following a diet with many restrictions, evaluation is important. Monitoring the diet can provide invaluable information on both nutrient levels and on habits associated with them. Thought patterns can be important (Appendix F). On return visits, discussion should revolve around information the clients have recorded.

Clients should be given an opportunity for self-evaluation. This allows them to review their adherence to the diet and possibly go back and change behaviors where problems occur. The following is a checklist of points clients can evaluate:

_____ 1. Although dietary changes have been drastic, I have learned to conform to the changes and, where necessary, adjust my life style accordingly.

_____ 2. I was able to tackle problem situations gradually.

_____ 3. Social occasions always pose problems. However, by looking at the situation and preparing for it, coping is easier.

_____ 4. My family is involved with my dietary changes.

_____ 5. My family provides needed positive reinforcement.

For nutrition counselors, evaluation of their own progress is equally valuable. They can use the following checklist:

____ 1. Did assessment point to areas where adherence to the diet could be a problem?

____ 2. Did the protein-modified eating pattern take into consideration the client's life style as much as was realistically possible?

____ 3. Were the strategies used to increase adherence to the protein-modified regimen carried out efficiently?

____ 4. Were appropriate verbal and nonverbal interviewing skills used when dietary changes caused difficulties?

____ 5. Where might changes might be made?_____
_____
_____
_____
_____
_____

____ 6. Where adherence to the protein-modified eating pattern was a problem did I use appropriate counseling skills?

____ 7. Where might changes have been made?_____
_____
_____
_____
_____
_____

____ 8. What general changes would I make in the next counseling interview with a similar client on a protein-modified diet?_____
_____
_____
_____
_____
_____

These checklists can be used as guides. Clients and counselors also might want to develop their own checklist for evaluating the counseling session.

Adherence Tool 7–1 Monitoring Device

Time	Protein-Containing Food	Amount	Source	Essential Amino Acids*

Daily Record of Foods Containing Protein

*If food contains all essential amino acids, place an X in the final column.

Review of Chapter 7
(Answers in Appendix I)

1. List four factors associated with inappropriate eating behaviors when following a protein-modified eating pattern:
   a. _____
   b. _____
   c. _____
   d. _____
2. Identify four possible nutrients that should be identified as to baseline intake:
   a. _____
   b. _____
   c. _____
   d. _____

Adherence Tool 7–2 Informational Device

Client Diet Base and One-Day Menu

My diet should contain _____ grams of protein per day.
Examples of foods containing all essential amino acids:

Meats	Fish	Milk
Poultry	Eggs	Cheese

Examples of foods lacking one or more essential amino acids:

Breads	Fruits	Cereals
Vegetables	Gelatin	

Essential amino acids are:

Histidine	Threonine
Isoleucine	Tryptophan
Leucine	Valine
Lysine	

Plan one day's menu using protein-containing foods:

Breakfast	Lunch	Dinner	Snacks

3. List four strategies to treat inappropriate eating behaviors associated with protein-modified patterns:

a. _____

b. _____

c. _____

d. _____

4. The following is an exercise to help in applying the ideas just discussed:

> John is a 31-year-old minister who eats all of his meals at home except for a few social gatherings. His major problem is his wife's reluctance to help him modify his diet because she feels there are too many restrictions. Explain what you would do, and why, to change the wife's feelings about the diet. (Don't presume the significant other's behavior will change)

---

5. List five possible questions a counselor might raise in helping the client evaluate progress:

   a. _____
   b. _____
   c. _____
   d. _____
   e. _____

6. List five questions to review in evaluating counselor progress:

   a. _____
   b. _____
   c. _____
   d. _____
   e. _____

NOTES

1. Food and Nutrition Board, *Recommended Dietary Allowances* (Washington, D.C.: National Academy of Sciences, National Research Council, 1980), 43.

2. Helen S. Mitchell et al., *Nutrition in Health and Disease*, 16th ed. (Philadelphia: J.B. Lippincott Company, 1976), 41.

3. Food and Nutrition Board, *Recommended Allowances,* 46–51.

4. Eleanor Noss Whitney and Eva May Nunnelley Hamilton, *Understanding Nutrition* (St. Paul, Minn.: West Publishing Company, 1981), 113.

5. Mitchell et al., *Nutrition,* 446–447.

6. Ibid.

7. Ibid.

SUGGESTED READINGS

Books

A Guide to Protein Controlled Diets. Los Angeles: California Dietetic Association.

American Dietetic Association. *Handbook of Clinical Dietetics.* New Haven, Conn.: Yale University Press, 1981.

Berlyne, Geoffrey M., ed. *Nutrition in Renal Disease.* Baltimore: The Williams and Wilkins Co., 1968.

Goodhart, Robert S., and Shils, Maurice E. *Modern Nutrition in Health and Disease.* Philadelphia: Lea and Febiger, 1980.

Hansen, Ginny L., ed. *Caring for Patients with Chronic Renal Disease.* Philadelphia: J.B. Lippincott Co., 1972.

Kidney Foundation of Illinois. *Fun with Food for Dialysis Patients.* Chicago: Illinois Council on Renal Nutrition, 1977.

Krause, Marie V., and Mahan, L. Kathleen. *Food, Nutrition and Diet Therapy,* 6th rev. ed. Philadelphia: W.B. Saunders Company, 1979.

Low Protein Diets Made Simple. Loma Linda, Calif.: University Medical Center, Dietary Department.

Spritzer, M.E. *A Renal Failure Diet Manual Utilizing the Food Exchange System.* Springfield, Ill.: Charles C Thomas Publishers, 1976.

U.S. Public Health Service. *Living with End-Stage Renal Failure, A Book for Patients.* Washington, D.C.: U.S. Government Printing Office, 1976.

Articles

Anderson, Carl F. "Nutritional Therapy for Adults with Renal Disease." *Journal of the American Medical Association* 223(1973):68–72.

Bailey, George L., and Sullivan, Nancy R. "Selected-Protein Diet in Terminal Uremia." *Journal of the American Dietetic Association* 52(1968):125–129.

Burton, Benjamin T. "Current Concepts of Nutrition and Diet in Diseases of the Kidney." *Journal of the American Dietetic Association* 65(1974):623–626.

Cohodes, Aaron. "A Better Care Aim of Dialysis Network." *Hospitals* 49(1975):44–48.

Giovannetti, S., and Maggiore, Q. "A Low-Nitrogen Diet with Proteins of High Biological Value for Severe Uraemia." *Lancet* 1(1964):1000–1003.

Kopple, Joel D., and Swendseid, Marian E. "Nitrogen Balance and Plasma Amino Acid Levels in Uremic Patients Fed an Essential Amino Acid Diet." *American Journal of Clinical Nutrition* 27(1974):806–812.

———. "Histidine Deficiency Anemia in Renal Failure." *Clinical Research* 21(1973):266.

Landsman, Melanie K. "The Patient with Chronic Renal Failure." *Annals of Internal Medicine* 82(1975):268–270.

Niwa, Toyoo. "Plasma Level and Transfer Capacity of Thiamin in Patients Undergoing Long-Term Hemodialysis." *American Journal of Clinical Nutrition* 28(1975):1105–1109.

Santopietro, Mary and Charles S. "Meeting the Emotional Needs of Hemodialysis Patients and Their Spouses." *American Journal of Nursing* 75(1975):629–632.

Vetter, Laura, and Shapiro, Ronald. "An Approach to Dietary Management of the Patient with Renal Disease." *Journal of the American Dietetic Association* 66(1975):158–162.

Counseling for Low-Sodium Eating Patterns

Objectives for Chapter 8

1. Identify factors that lead to inappropriate eating behaviors associated with sodium-modified regimens.
2. Identify important steps in the assessment of a baseline diet for clients following a low-sodium eating pattern.
3. Identify strategies to treat inappropriate eating behaviors associated with sodium-modified patterns.
4. Generate strategies to use in facilitating problem solving for clients who are following low-sodium patterns.
5. Identify elements necessary for both client and counselor evaluation.
6. Recommend dietary adherence tools for clients on sodium-modified eating patterns.

8

INAPPROPRIATE EATING BEHAVIORS

Diets modified in sodium content may be extremely difficult for most clients with whom nutrition counselors must deal. Salt is used as a flavoring agent in nearly every food. Altering such dietary habits means drastic changes for most clients.

Counselors frequently hear the complaint, "I really miss familiar flavors" or "Everything I eat tastes like sawdust." For unconscious salters (those who salt without tasting), the true flavors of foods may never have come through. They gradually will be able to discover the natural flavors in foods through treatments suggested in this chapter.

The new eating pattern will limit their food options because most commercial products are very high in sodium. With the trend to the use of prepackaged commercial meals and other products, clients on a low-sodium regimen are left with fewer choices.

This limitation has led to many alterations in old eating habits. Clients not only must change what they usually eat but also must become accustomed to a new and foreign range of food flavors.

The food industry, in an effort to assist these persons, has developed a variety of low-salt products. However, these do generate comments such as, "You expect me to eat this low-sodium soup? It's terrible." Another complaint is that some salt substitutes leave a bitter aftertaste. Objections to commercial low-sodium products constitute a recurring problem for nutrition counselors.

ASSESSMENT OF EATING BEHAVIORS

For clients who must follow a low-sodium diet, a baseline assessment is crucial. Such regimens require changes in many foods individuals routinely and even unconsciously consume. Identifying when, where, with whom, and how much sodium is consumed can be of great benefit in helping to reduce salt intake patterns. The format in Table 8–1 can be used to collect baseline data.

In collecting this information the clients are self-monitoring their sodium intake. Before actually using the form, clients should be asked simply to observe their general behaviors involving sodium consumption, i.e., salting before tasting. They should be told which basic foods are high in sodium.

During the baseline data collection clients actually begin counting sodium intake occurrences, along with related information indicated in the form. These guidelines can be of help:

1. The form must be portable and readily available for recording.
2. The clients must be familiar enough with high-sodium foods to record all occurrences of the target behavior (sodium intake).

Table 8–1 Sodium Intake Information

Food	Amount		Time	Place	Who Present
	In Cooking	At Table			

3. The clients should record the data as the behaviors occur.
4. The clients always should keep written records—memory is not adequate for baseline data collection.[1]

During this period, some changes in behavior may occur automatically. That will make the nutrition counselors' job that much easier. Unfortunately, not all clients will respond with behavior changes during this time and will need guidance in the treatment phase. Counselors also should emphasize to the clients that treatment interventions should be started after, not before, the baseline data collection.

One important aspect during data collection is the clients' increasing awareness of and attention to sodium intake. For example, during a meal they may become conscious of salting food before tasting. They also should elicit help from friends and family. There are many ways family members can delicately and supportively word their attempts to point out excessive use of sodium.

The clients never should allow the recordkeeping to become a punishment, so counselors must help find ways to reinforce this function positively.

Clients should be aware of how important the baseline data are in identifying types of foods, amounts, and related factors—information that will improve their adherence to the dietary pattern. At this point they might well ask, "How long should I keep baseline data?" The reply depends on several factors:

1. The data collection should continue for at least one week, since the intake of sodium occurs daily.
2. It would be best to gather data for two weeks if an initial review reveals large variations in sodium intake from one day to the next.
3. Data should be recorded long enough to provide a good estimate of when in a day the largest amounts of sodium are consumed.
4. The data gathering can end when clients and counselors are satisfied that the actual patterns and frequencies of sodium intake are shown by the records that have been kept.[2]

Clients also may wonder when they will know that a stable baseline has been reached. Watson and Tharp provide the following guidelines:

1. It is rare to get a stable baseline in less than one week. It generally should run at least one "normal" week and should go beyond three or four weeks only rarely.
2. The greater the variation from day to day, the longer it will take to get a stable baseline.

3. Clients should be asked to be sure the period during which the data were gathered is representative of their usual life style.[3]

In helping clients fill out the recording form, counselors should ask:

1. Are the categories to be recorded defined specifically?
2. Are both sodium intakes and related factors recorded?
3. Will the form always be present during times of food consumption?
4. Is the format simple and not punishing or intimidating?
5. Is it possible to reinforce the recordkeeping positively?[4]

TREATMENT STRATEGIES

Before providing treatment strategies, counselors should identify a general problem that can be solved first. Along with the statement of that problem, inappropriate regular eating patterns should be identified. Clients should be asked to help discover possible solutions, with the counselors providing expertise by drawing from the strategies described next.

Tailoring and staging strategies help focus the dietary pattern on the clients' special needs. Behavior change is necessary for social occasions and for the routine alterations in eating style that the regimen requires.

Most nutrition counselors provide lists of standard do's and dont's for low-sodium eating patterns. This does not allow for individualizing eating patterns to meet each client's needs. The counselors tailor the eating pattern to the clients, first by carefully studying the baseline information. Attention must be paid not only to consumption of sodium but also to other factors that are associated with its intake. If clients have a favorite high-sodium food, the counselors can discuss how it might be incorporated to meet a 2,000-milligram sodium limit, cautioning that other foods containing sodium may have to be eliminated or reduced in amounts. Compromises as to the amount of the favorite foods allowed should be discussed as well.

In tailoring, the counselors should point out which foods on the diet record qualify for the sodium-restricted eating pattern. Foods the clients routinely eat and like should be discussed and the reasons for full acceptance, curtailment, or elimination explained. Any and all positive aspects of the low-sodium eating pattern should be built up.

Staging the diet can be a crucial factor in maintaining adherence over time. It is very tempting for counselors to hand clients a list of foods high in sodium and send them on their way complaining about how they never will be able to follow the diet.

In beginning the staging process there are two simple rules:

1. It can never begin too low.
2. The steps upward can never be too small.

As the interviews progress, these rules should be individualized for each client. If the sessions move too slowly, the counselors can move up a step or discuss fewer steps.

Staging helps clients feel that changes are easy and, therefore, that their chances for success are increased. Staging also can help in analysis of the component parts of these situations.

An alternative to this approach is to stage the dietary restrictions for sodium, with the clients slowly adjusting to sets of restrictions. One way is to start with the group of foods easiest to begin using in low-sodium form. This enables clients to achieve success with the initial group. The baseline data can be used to prepare lists in consultation with the clients.

A common experience in following staging schedules is the plateau. Week after week the clients may make excellent progress, then suddenly stop. Moving up through all of those previous steps may have seemed so easy but now a new one—the same size as all the rest—seems very difficult. The easiest way to continue to progress is to subdivide that difficult step. If this does not help, the counselors should try increasing the reinforcement.

Many clients will confide to the practitioners that they are guilty of cheating. This occurs when they take the reinforcers even though they have not achieved a particular step. In such cases, the counselors must redesign the staged schedule so clients can be reinforced at a level they find achievable.

Some clients complain that they are losing the willpower to follow the low-sodium diet. They may experience this in two ways:

1. They cannot get started. Counselors and clients may not have set the initial step low enough. This can be resolved by moving to a lower step.
2. They may have started but insist that they see no progress. In that case, smaller steps are necessary.

In changing eating behaviors it is important for counselors to review with the clients the following sequence: antecedent-behavior-consequence. The counselors begin to identify antecedents (events that precede a be-

Table 8-2 Chart of Spices That Can Substitute for Salt

SPICE	APPETIZER	SOUP	MEAT and EGGS	FISH & POULTRY	SAUCES	VEGETABLES	SALAD & DRESSING	DESSERTS
ALLSPICE	Cocktail Meatballs	Pot Au Feu	Hamsteak	Oyster Stew	Barbecue	Eggplant Creole	Cottage Cheese Dressing	Apple Tapioca Pudding
BASIL	Cheese Stuffed Celery	Manhattan Clam Chowder	Ragout of Beef	Shrimp Creole	Spaghetti	Stewed Tomatoes	Russian Dressing	
BAY LEAF	Pickled Beets	Vegetable Soup	Lamb Stew	Simmered Chicken	Bordelaise	Boiled New Potatoes	Tomato Juice Dressing	
CARAWAY Seed	Mild Cheese Spreads		Sauerbraten		Beef a la Mode Sauce	Cabbage Wedges		
CINNAMON	Cranberry Juice	Fruit Soup	Pork Chops	Sweet and Sour Fish	Butter Sauce for Squash	Sweet Potato Croquettes	Stewed Fruit Salad	Chocolate Pudding
CAYENNE	Deviled Eggs	Oyster Stew	Barbecued Beef	Poached Salmon Hollandaise	Bearnaise	Cooked Greens	Tuna Fish Salad	
CELERY Salt and Seed	Ham Spread (Salt)	Cream of Celery (Seed)	Meat Loaf (Seed)	Chicken Croquettes (Salt)	Celery Sauce (Seed)	Cauliflower (Salt)	Cole Slaw (Seed)	
CHERVIL	Fish Dips	Cream Soup	Omelet	Chicken Saute	Vegetable Sauce	Peas Francaise	Caesar Salad	
CHILI Powder	Seafood Cocktail Sauce	Pepper Pot	Chili con Carne	Arroz con Pollo	Meat Gravy	Corn Mexicali	Chili French Dressing	
CLOVES	Fruit Punch	Mulligatawny	Boiled Tongue	Baked Fish	Sauce Madeira	Candied Sweet Potatoes		Stewed Pears
CURRY Powder	Curried Shrimp	Cream of Mushroom	Curry of Lamb	Chicken Hash	Orientale or Indienne	Creamed Vegetables	Curried Mayonnaise	
DILL Seed	Cottage Cheese	Split Pea	Grilled Lamb Steak	Drawn Butter for Shellfish	Dill Sauce for Fish or Chicken	Peas and Carrots	Sour Cream Dressing	
GARLIC Salt or Powder	Clam Dip	Vegetable Soup	Roast Lamb	Bouillabaisse	Garlic Butter	Eggs and Tomato Casserole	Tomato and Cucumber Salad	
GINGER	Broiled Grapefruit	Bean Soup	Dust lightly over Steak	Roast Chicken	Cocktail	Buttered Beets	Cream Dressing for Ginger Pears	Stewed Dried Fruits

	Quiche Lorraine	Petite Marmite	Veal Fricasse	Fish Stew	Creole	Succotash	Fruit Salad	Cottage Pudding
MACE	Quiche Lorraine							
MARJORAM	Fruit Punch Cup	Onion Soup	Roast Lamb	Salmon Loaf	Brown	Eggplant	Mixed Green Salad	
MINT	Fruit Cup	Sprinkle over Split Pea	Veal Roast	Cold Fish	Lamb	Green Peas	Cottage Cheese Salad	Ambrosia
MUSTARD Powdered Dry	Ham Spread	Lobster Bisque	Virginia Ham	Deviled Crab	Cream Sauce for Fish	Baked Beans	Egg Salad	Gingerbread Cookies
NUTMEG	Chopped Oysters	Cream DuBarry	Salisbury Steak	Southern Fried Chicken	Mushroom	Glazed Carrots	Sweet Salad Dressing	Sprinkle over Vanilla Ice Cream
ONION Powder, Salt, Flakes and Instant Minced Onion	Avocado Spread (Powder)	Consommes (Flakes)	Meat Loaf (Instant Minced Onion)	Fried Shrimp (Salt)	Tomato (Powder)	Broiled Tomatoes (Salt)	Vinaigrette Dressing (Instant Minced Onion)	
OREGANO	Sharp Cheese Spread	Beef Soup	Swiss Steak	Court Bouillon	Spaghetti	Boiled Onions	Sea Food	
PAPRIKA	Creamed Seafood	Creamed Soup	Hungarian Goulash	Oven Fried Chicken	Paprika Cream	Baked Potato	Cole Slaw	
PARSLEY Flakes	Cheese Balls	Cream of Asparagus	Irish Lamb Stew	Broiled Mackerel	Chasseur	French Fried Potatoes	Tossed Green Salad	
ROSEMARY	Deviled Eggs	Mock Turtle	Lamb Loaf	Chicken a la King	Cheese	Sauteed Mushrooms	Meat Salad	
SAGE	Cheese Spreads	Consomme	Cold Roast Beef	Poultry Stuffing	Duck	Brussels Sprouts	Herbed French Dressing	
SAVORY	Liver Paste	Lentil Soup	Scrambled Eggs	Chicken Loaf	Fish	Beets	Red Kidney Bean Salad	
TARRAGON	Mushrooms a la Greque	Snap Bean Soup	Marinated Lamb or Beef	Lobster	Green	Buttered Broccoli	Chicken Salad	
THYME	Artichokes	Clam Chowder	Use sparingly in Fricasses	Poultry Stuffing	Bordelaise	Lightly on Sauteed Mushrooms	Tomato Aspic	

Source: Reprinted from *How to Stay on a Low-Calorie, Low-Sodium Diet* with permission of the American Spice Trade Association, © 1980.

havior) by asking the clients to think about the following questions as they relate to an eating occurrence:

1. What were the physical circumstances? (i.e., was the client surrounded by large tables of food?)
2. What was the social setting?
3. What was the behavior of others?
4. What did you think or say to yourself?[5]

The client should be asked to collect data related to antecedents.

In changing eating behaviors, one tactic is to lengthen the chain of events before partaking of a desired item such as high-sodium cheese. By pausing before eating, immediate gratification is delayed and the behavior eventually may not occur at all. It also may be possible to interrupt the chain by identifying an early link; a discontinuance or prolonged pause at that point may prevent the inappropriate behavior from occurring. The events also may be scrambled so that the eventual behavior never is reached.

Another strategy is to provide good substitutions for salt—other flavoring agents such as spices, herbs, fruit juices, etc.—as proposed in Table 8–2.

The average sodium content of all spices is less than one milligram per teaspoon. The spice highest in sodium is parsley flakes, which contain not quite six milligrams per teaspoon. In comparison, one gram of salt contains 2,300 milligrams of sodium.

The importance of reading labels carefully should be stressed because some spices are prepared in combination with salt. Anyone on a low-sodium diet should avoid the spice-salt combination products. Table 8–3 indicates the sodium content of spices prepared without salt.

Social occasions can present special problems. The clients can begin to learn to cope with such situations by collecting data on what types of reinforcers maintain their eating of high-sodium foods during social events. The same reinforcer that maintains an undesired eating behavior can be used to strengthen appropriate conduct. For example:

CLIENT at a party: "Boy, do those salty chips look good. But I know that they aren't on my diet. Over here, though, are some fresh vegetables. They look just as good and are on my diet. I feel really good about myself after eating them and I haven't cheated on my diet."

In helping to maintain a low-sodium diet it may be helpful to keep a list of positive reinforcers. Watson and Tharp provide a set of questions clients might be asked when making a list of positive reinforcers:

1. What kinds of low-sodium foods do you like to eat?
2. What are your major interests?

Table 8–3 Sodium Content of Spices

Spice	Milligrams/ teaspoon	Spice	Milligrams/ teaspoon
Allspice	1.4		
Basil Leaves	0.4	Nutmeg	0.2
Bay Leaves	0.3	Onion Powder	0.8
Caraway Seed	0.4	Oregano	0.3
Cardamon Seed	0.2	Paprika	0.4
Celery Seed	4.1	Parsley Flakes	5.9
Cinnamon	0.2	Pepper, Black	0.2
Cloves	4.2	Pepper, Chili	0.2
Coriander Seed	0.3	Pepper, Red	0.2
Cumin Seed	2.6	Pepper, White	0.2
Curry Powder	1.0	Poppy Seed	0.2
Dill Seed	0.2	Rosemary Leaves	0.5
Fennel Seed	1.9	Sage	0.1
Garlic Powder	0.1	Savory	0.3
Ginger	0.5	Sesame Seed	0.6
Mace	1.3	Tarragon	1.0
Marjoram	1.3	Thyme	1.2
Mustard Powder	0.1	Turmeric	0.2

Source: Reprinted from *Low-Sodium Spice Tips* with permission of the American Spice Trade Association, © 1980.

3. What are your hobbies?
4. What people do you like to be with?
5. What do you like to do with these people?
6. What do you do for fun, for enjoyment?
7. What do you do to relax?
8. What do you do to get away from it all?
9. What makes you feel good?
10. What would be a nice present to receive?
11. What kinds of things are important to you?
12. What would you buy if you had an extra five dollars? Ten dollars? Fifty dollars?
13. What behaviors do you perform every day?
14. Are there any behaviors that you usually perform instead of the target behavior?
15. What would you hate to lose?
16. Of the things you do every day, what would you hate to give up?[6]

Additional questions could be constructed. Determining the best reinforcers will depend upon each individual client.

Before choosing a reinforcer, counselors should consider how closely
the consequence is tailored individually to meet a client's needs and desires.
The reinforcer must be manageable from the client's point of view. It also
must be contingent upon performance of the desired behavior—eating low-
sodium foods. The reinforcer should be strong enough to help in changing
behavior.

The next step in helping to alter behavior is to set up a contract (Exhibit
8–1, for a woman client) that should specify the following:

1. Stages of the change in eating habits
2. Kinds of reinforcers to be gained at each step
3. Self-agreement to make gaining those reinforcers contingent
   upon changing eating behavior involving high-sodium foods.[7]

Ideally, a contract should be written and signed and should specify each
detail of dietary change. Each element of this intervention plan should be
very specific. A plan—a written contract—will help clients in those inev-
itable moments of weakness.

In selecting reinforcers, it is important that they are within the realm of
possibility or are readily accessible. They also should be potent. For example, buying clothes is not a potent reinforcer if the client does not enjoy
doing it. The clients should be told to use "intuition" or estimate potency.

Exhibit 8–1 Contract for a Sodium-Modified Diet

I agree to carry out each of the following steps and supply each reinforcer listed as each
step is achieved:

Steps	Reinforcer
1. Eliminate salting before tasting	Read a new cookbook
2. Slowly eat unsalted foods to allow detection of true flavors	Buy a new scarf
3. Add new spices to foods in place of salt	Buy a new pair of shoes

Signed: _____

Cosigned (counselor): _____

Date: _____

The counselors' own data, collected during intervention, can indicate whether or not the chosen reinforcer is sufficiently powerful. Reinforcement of a desired eating behavior should occur immediately after the clients have performed it. The longer reinforcement is delayed, the less effective it will be.

If it is impossible to deliver reinforcement immediately, token reinforcers can be appropriate. A token is a symbolic reinforcer because it can be converted into real reinforcement. Tokens include money, poker chips, gold stars, checkmarks, and ticket punches. A point system also can be used (this one is for a woman client; reinforcers for men and youngsters will vary):

One token..one new blouse
Two tokens ....two new blouses
Three tokens ....a new dress
Four tokens...a new suit

Reinforcement can be increased as a new eating behavior becomes more frequent. This provides additional incentives for continuing self-modification.

One particular reinforcer should not be overused or clients will become satiated by it. In other words, a specific reward loses its reinforcing quality through overrepetition.

A reinforcer that punishes someone else should not be used. For example, if a married woman client uses money to buy a dress as a reinforcer, the counselor must be sure the husband is in agreement.

The discussion and dispensing of reinforcers can and should involve the family directly. If the family members are aware of potent reinforcers, they can help in dispensing them at opportune times.

With low-sodium diets, nutrition forms the base upon which all treatment strategies hang. The Food and Nutrition Board has not established a Recommended Dietary Allowance for sodium. However, it does provide an estimate of daily minimal sodium intakes for children of approximately 58 milligrams.[8] The board adds that adults can maintain sodium balance with an intake of little more than the children's minimal requirement.

Mitchell and her coworkers describe three levels of sodium restriction:

1. 2,000 to 3,000 milligrams of sodium per day constitutes a mild restriction.
2. 1,000 to 2,000 milligrams of sodium is a moderate restriction.
3. Fewer than 1,000 milligrams imposes a severe restriction.[9]

It is possible to provide a rough guide for the natural sodium content of foods that are grown or produced and processed without the addition of sodium. Mitchell and her coworkers offer the following:

8 oz. milk	=	120 mg. of sodium
1 oz. meat	=	25 mg. of sodium
1 egg	=	70 mg. of sodium
½ cup vegetable	=	9 mg. of sodium
½ cup fruit	=	2 mg. of sodium
1 slice of bread	=	5 mg. of sodium
1 teaspoon of fat*	=	0 mg. of sodium

In some cases it is necessary to convert milliequivalents (mEq.) to milligrams of sodium. One milliequivalent of sodium is 23 milligrams, the gram-atomic weight. A diet prescription of 40 milliequivalents of sodium is equal to 920 milligrams of sodium (23 mg. $\times$ 40 mEq. = 920 mg.). Sodium chloride contains 39.3 percent sodium. This means that 10 grams of salt contain 3.93 grams of sodium (10 g. $\times$ .393 = 3.93 g.).

As noted earlier, the sodium-restricted diet is probably the most difficult of all food therapies for clients. Ethnic foods can pose particular problems. Soy sauce and monosodium glutamate, often found in oriental cookery, are extremely high in sodium. Jewish clients who follow their dietary laws of heavily salting meats before cooking (koshering) will need help in modifying their eating behaviors. Southern cookery includes bacon and salt pork, both of which are high in sodium. Greek clients and those from the Near East use heavily salted olives as an accompaniment to many meals.

EVALUATION OF BEHAVIORS

In monitoring sodium intake during the dietary intervention, clients can use a form like that in Table 8-1 (supra). Counselors should review the form with the clients during follow-up visits.

The evaluation of progress on a low-sodium diet can involve allowing the clients to respond to the following:

_____ 1. My goal was reached in eliminating extremely high-sodium foods.
_____ 2. My eating patterns have changed because of reinforcers.
_____ 3. The circumstances involving my high-sodium eating behaviors have changed.

---

*1 teaspoon of unsalted butter contains ¼ mg. of sodium, 1 teaspoon of regular butter to which salt has been added contains 50 mg. of sodium.

____ 4. Social occasions are less of a problem now than when I began my eating pattern.

____ 5. My family provides needed positive reinforcement.

The counselors' checklist, which can be modified to fit specific cases, includes the following points:

____ 1. Was assessment of baseline sodium intake adequate to help in staging the eating pattern?

____ 2. Did each staged section of the dietary instruction include attention to the client's previous life style?

____ 3. Were strategies to promote adherence to the low-sodium eating pattern carried out efficiently?

____ 4. Did I use appropriate verbal and nonverbal interviewing skills when confronting the client with necessary dietary changes?

____ 5. What might I have done differently?_____
_____
_____
_____
_____
_____

____ 6. Where dietary adherence was a problem, did I use appropriate counseling skills?

____ 7. What improvements might have been made?_____
_____
_____
_____
_____
_____

____ 8. What general changes would I make in the next counseling interview with a similar client on a sodium-modified eating pattern?
_____
_____
_____
_____
_____
_____

This evaluation process is crucial to eventual success for both client and counselor. Additional factors can be considered:

Client	Counselor
1. _____	1. _____
2. _____	2. _____
3. _____	3. _____
4. _____	4. _____
5. _____	5. _____

Adherence Tool 8–1 Monitoring Device

Daily Food Record with Emphasis on Sodium Intake					
Time	Food Eaten	Amount	Low in Na+*	Moderate in Na+*	High in Na+*

*Place an X in the column to indicate whether the food is high, moderate, or low in sodium.

Adherence Tool 8–2 Informational Device

Spices for Low-Sodium Diets

Spices for Use with Meats:

Dill seed for fish or chicken sauces
Garlic powder for bouillabaisse
Ginger for roast chicken
Mace for fish stew
Marjoram for salmon loaf

Mint for veal or lamb roast
Mustard for cream sauce on fish
Nutmeg for southern fried chicken
Oregano for Swiss steak
Rosemary for chicken à la king
Savory for chicken loaf
Tarragon for marinated beef
Thyme for clam chowder

Spices for Use with Vegetables:

Allspice for eggplant creole
Basil for stewed tomatoes
Bay leaf for boiled new potatoes
Caraway seed for cabbage wedges
Cinnamon for sweet potatoes
Celery seed for cauliflower
Chili powder for Mexican-style corn

Cloves for candied sweet potatoes
Curry for creamed vegetables
Dill seed for peas and carrots
Garlic for stewed tomatoes
Ginger for beets
Mace for succotash
Mint for green peas
Powdered dry mustard for baked beans
Nutmeg for glazed carrots
Rosemary for sauteed mushrooms
Sage for Brussels sprouts
Savory for beets
Tarragon for broccoli
Thyme lightly on sauteed mushrooms

Plan menus for three meals. The menus should be low in sodium and should use the spices suggested above. Choose spices you think you and your family would enjoy.

BREAKFAST	LUNCH	DINNER

Review of Chapter 8

(Answers in Appendix I)

1. List four factors that lead to inappropriate eating behaviors associated with sodium-modified patterns.

   a. _____

   b. _____

   c. _____

   d. _____

2. Identify three important steps in the assessment of a baseline diet for clients following a low-sodium regimen.

   a. _____
   _____

   b. _____
   _____

   c. _____
   _____

3. List four strategies to use in treating problems associated with eating patterns low in sodium.

   a. _____
   _____

   b. _____
   _____

   c. _____
   _____

   d. _____
   _____

4. Mrs. B. is 40 years old and has just been placed on a low-sodium diet. She has collected baseline information. She says she has tried and failed to follow a low-sodium diet previously. She loves cheese and cold cuts. What other facts would be beneficial to know? Based on hypothetical answers to those facts, what strategies would you recommend to solve her problems with low-sodium eating patterns?

   _____
   _____
   _____
   _____
   _____
   _____
   _____
   _____
   _____

_____
_____
_____
_____
_____
_____
_____
_____
_____
_____
_____

5. What questions might you cover with the client to help determine how well the diet was followed?

  a. _____
     _____

  b. _____
     _____

  c. _____
     _____

  d. _____
     _____

6. What questions might you ask to evaluate yourself as a counselor?

  a. _____
     _____

  b. _____
     _____

  c. _____
     _____

  d. _____
     _____

NOTES

1. David L. Watson and Roland G. Tharp, *Self-Directed Behavior: Self-Modification for Personal Adjustment* (Monterey, Calif.: Brooks/Cole Publishing Company, 1972), 85–89.

2. Ibid., 96–97.

3. Ibid., 97–98.

4. Ibid., 99.

5. Ibid., 148.

6. Ibid., 108.

7. Ibid., 117.

8. Food and Nutrition Board, *Recommended Dietary Allowances,* 9th ed. (Washington D.C.: National Academy of Sciences, National Research Council, 1980), 170.

9. Helen S. Mitchell et. al., *Nutrition in Health and Disease* (Philadelphia: J.B. Lippincott Company, 1976), 430.

SUGGESTED READINGS

Books

American Heart Association. *Your 500-Milligram Sodium Diet.* New York: American Heart Association, 1968.

———. *Your Mild Sodium-Restricted Diet.* New York: American Heart Association, 1969.

Bagg, E. *Cooking Without a Grain of Salt.* New York: Bantam Books, 1973.

Diet Committee of the San Francisco Heart Association. *Sodium in Medicines.* San Francisco: San Francisco Heart Association, 1973.

Dupuy, M.E., and Dupuy, B.J. *Fat-Controlled and Sodium-Restricted Cooking.* Garden City, N.Y.: Doubleday and Company, 1971.

Food and Nutrition Board. *The Use of Chemicals in Food Production, Processing, Storage and Distribution.* Washington, D.C.: National Academy of Sciences, National Research Council, 1973.

Goodhart, Robert S., and Shils, Maurice E. *Modern Nutrition in Health and Disease,* 6th rev. ed. Philadelphia: Lea and Febiger, 1980.

Julian, Desmond G. *Cardiology,* 3rd rev. ed. London: Bailliere Tindall, 1978.

National Research Council. *Sodium-Restricted Diets,* Publication no. 325. Washington, D.C.: National Academy of Sciences, 1954.

Payne, A.S., and Callahan, D. *The Low-Sodium, Fat-Controlled Cookbook,* 4th rev. ed. Boston: Little, Brown and Co., 1975.

Robinson, Corinne H., and Lawler, Marilyn R. *Normal and Therapeutic Nutrition,* 15th rev. ed. New York: Macmillan Publishing Co., Inc., 1977.

Salmon, Margaret B., and Quigley, Althea E. *Enjoying Your Restricted Diet.* Springfield, Ill.: Charles C Thomas, Publisher, 1972.

Articles

Altschul, A.M. "Salt Sensitivity in Experimental Animals and Man." *International Journal of Obesity* 5(1981): Supplement 1, 27–38.

Buccicone, Jenny, and McAllister, R.G. "Failure of Single Session Dietary Counseling to Reduce Salt Intake in Hypertensive Patients." *Southern Medical Journal* 70(1977):1436–1438.

Christakis, George, and Winston, Mary. "Nutritional Therapy in Acute Myocardial Infarction." *Journal of the American Dietetic Association* 63(1973):233–238.

Conn, Harold O. "Diuresis of Ascites: Fraught with or Free from Hazard." *Gastroenterology* 73(1977):619–621.

Dahl, Lewis K. "Salt and Hypertension." *American Journal of Clinical Nutrition* 25(1972):231–244.

Dustan, Harriet R.; Tarazi, Robert C.; and Bravo, Emmanuel L. "Diuretic and Diet Treatment of Hypertension." *Archives of Internal Medicine* 133(1974):1007–1013.

Faust, Halley S. "Effects of Drinking Water and Total Sodium Intake on Blood Pressure." *American Journal of Clinical Nutrition* 35(1982):1459–1467.

Gordon, Edgar S. "Dietary Problems in Hypertension." *Geriatrics* 29(1974):139–144.

Kawasaki, Terukazu. "The Effect of High Sodium and Low Sodium Intakes on Blood Pressure and Other Related Variables in Human Subjects with Idiopathic Hypertension." *American Journal of Medicine* 64(1978):193–198.

Kirkendall, Walter M. "The Effect of Dietary Sodium Chloride on Blood Pressure, Body Fluids, Electrolytes, Renal Function, and Serum Lipids of Normotensive Man." *Journal of Laboratory and Clinical Medicine* 87(1976):418–434.

Loggie, Jennifer M.H. "Renal Function and Diuretic Therapy in Infants and Children." *Journal of Pediatrics* 86(1975):485, 657, 825.

McNeely, George R., and Batterbee, Harold D. "High Sodium-Low Potassium Environment and Hypertension." *American Journal of Cardiology* 38(1976):768–785.

Morgan, T. "Hypertension Treated by Salt Restriction." *Lancet* 1(1978):227–230.

Newborg, Barbara. "Sodium Restricted Diet." *Archives of Internal Medicine* 123(1969):692–693.

Newburgh, L.H., and Reimer, Ann. "The Rationale and Administration of Low Sodium Diets." *Journal of the American Dietetic Association* 23(1947):1047–1051.

Siegel, Norman J., and Myketey, Nadia. "Sodium, Potassium and Calorie Contents of Some Commercial Beverages." *Clinical Pediatrics* 11(1972):482–483.

"Spice Measurements in Grams." *Journal of the American Dietetic Association* 62(1973):290.

Walker, W. Gordon. "Relation Between Blood Pressure and Renin, Renin Substrate, Angiotensin II; Aldosterone and Urinary Sodium and Potassium in 574 Ambulatory Subjects." *Hypertension* 1(1979):287–291.

Other Materials

American Heart Association. *Fold-Out Charts: Sodium Restricted Diet, 500 mg.* (1965); *Sodium Restricted Diet, 1,000 mg.* (1966), and *Sodium Restricted Diet, Mild Restriction* (1967). New York: American Heart Association.

Counseling for Liberal Bland Diets

Objectives for Chapter 9

1. Identify important areas on which to focus data collection for clients who must follow liberal bland diets.
2. List treatment strategies to combat inappropriate eating behaviors.
3. Generate an appropriate strategy to use in facilitating problem solving for clients on liberal bland diets.
4. Identify elements necessary for both client and counselor evaluations.
5. Recommend dietary adherence tools for clients on diets modified in consistency and texture.

9

INAPPROPRIATE EATING BEHAVIORS

Nutrition counselors with clients on a liberal bland diet in most cases face fewer problem situations than with other restricted regimens. In those other dietary patterns, several restrictions can involve many food categories.

Inappropriate eating behaviors can result from reluctance to avoid a few favorite foods. Clients may complain of having to give up coffee, other caffeinated beverages, and pepper. Frequent feedings may mean changes in a normal schedule, which can cause problems.

ASSESSMENT OF EATING BEHAVIORS

In assessing dietary patterns and behaviors before placing clients on a liberal bland diet, nutrition counselors should begin by reviewing food preferences and the number of meals eaten each day. This information may be collected in various ways. Clients might record it in diet records that indicate foods, amounts (if desired), and the times at which they are eaten. Less elaborate may be a checklist on which clients indicate food preferences, then separately describe the times of day at which they are eaten.

By looking at food preferences and times of eating, counselors can identify areas in which behavior change must occur.

Counseling on a liberal bland eating pattern centers on the person and on normal nutritional needs rather than on a special regimen. Regularity and frequency of meals, and moderation in eating habits, are important in long-term care. Examples of general questions to be asked in the assessment phase are:

1. What changes should the client make in the present dietary pattern to provide necessary calories and nutrients?
2. What changes must be made in eating habits?
3. How will the client implement the changes?
4. What changes will the client need to make in life style?
5. Who can help in making these changes?[1]

Discussion of these actual or potential problem areas can form the basis for the development of treatment.

TREATMENT STRATEGIES

Two important strategies can be used to help clients overcome problems with a bland dietary pattern.

One strategy involves tailoring the eating pattern to the clients' life style. If they foresee general problems with eating more frequent and smaller meals, a time can be worked out most favorable for doing so. When they have mastered adding a chosen food at a new time of day, new times to add additional meals should be sought.

Throughout the second strategy, staging—the frequency of meals and tailoring by choosing favorite foods—the clients should have other family members present to learn about the new dietary modifications. The members should be shown how they can positively reinforce appropriate eating behaviors.

Nutrition is extremely important for clients who must follow a bland eating pattern. The American Dietetic Association (ADA) makes special recommendations for such persons in the treatment of chronic duodenal ulcer disease.[2] The ADA indicates that the rationale for use of chemically and mechanically nonirritating foods is not sufficiently supported by scientific evidence. Spices, condiments, and highly seasoned foods have not been shown to irritate the gastric mucosa but some items do: black pepper, chili powder, caffeine, coffee, tea, cocoa, alcohol, and drugs.

The benefits of milk in ulcer disease also are questionable. While milk does relieve duodenal ulcer pain, its acid-neutralizing effect is slight and its acid-producing effect could outweigh its buffering benefit. Research also indicates that fruit skins, lettuce, nuts, and celery, when masticated and mixed with saliva, do not scrape or irritate duodenal ulcers.[3,4]

Scientific investigation does support the validity of frequent small feedings for patients with duodenal ulcer disease.[5] The ADA also recommends individualizing the diet plan to include specific food intolerances, living patterns, life styles, work hours, and education. As with all meal patterns, the recommended dietary allowances should be kept in mind.

EVALUATION OF BEHAVIORS

Monitoring devices are used to collect baseline data. (See Adherence Tool 9–1 later in this chapter.) A food preference checklist may show changes from the baseline.

Each client should be asked to evaluate progress:

_____ 1. The bland eating pattern has been integrated into my current life style.

_____ 2. Each step in dietary change to meet the restrictions of the bland eating pattern has been met with little difficulty and with success.

_____ 3. My family provides needed positive reinforcement.

This checklist can be added to or modified by clients and counselors working together.

The practitioners also can formulate topics to evaluate the counseling sessions:

_____ 1. Was assessment of baseline for food preferences and frequency of eating adequate to help in staging the dietary pattern?

_____ 2. Did staging the dietary pattern take into account the client's previous life style?

_____ 3. Were strategies to promote adherence to the bland dietary pattern carried out efficiently?

_____ 4. Did I use appropriate verbal and nonverbal interviewing skills when confronting the client with necessary dietary changes?

_____ 5. What might I have done differently?

_____ 6. Where dietary adherence to the bland diet was a problem, did I use appropriate counseling skills?

_____ 7. What improvements might have been made?

_____
_____
_____
_____
_____
_____

_____ 8. What general changes would I make in the next counseling interview with a similar client following a bland eating pattern?

_____
_____
_____
_____
_____
_____

Any other factors that could be beneficial to the counselors can be added. Other elements that might be considered in both client and counselor evaluation include:

Client	Counselor
1. _____	1. _____
2. _____	2. _____
3. _____	3. _____
4. _____	4. _____
5. _____	5. _____

Review of Chapter 9
(Answers in Appendix I)

1. Identify two important areas on which to focus data collection for clients who must follow bland eating patterns.

   a. _____
   _____

   b. _____
   _____

Adherence Tool 9–1 Monitoring Device

Food Frequency Chart				
Food	Number of Times *Day*	*Week*	*Seldom Eat*	*Kind*
Milk				
Cheese, Cheddar				
Cheese, Cottage				
Yogurt				
Ice Cream, Pudding				
Eggs				
Fish				
Chicken, Turkey				
Beef				
Veal, Lamb, Pork (fresh)				
Luncheon meats, Wieners				
Dried Beans, Peas				
Peanut Butter				
Bacon, Salt Pork, Ham, Sausage				
Butter, Margarine				
Cooking Fat, Oil				
Salad Dressing				
Mayonnaise				
Orange, Grapefruit, or Juice				
Tomato Juice				
Fruit (raw)				
Fruit (canned)				
Green Vegetables (raw)				
Green Vegetables (canned)				
Yellow Vegetables (raw)				
Yellow Vegetables (canned)				
Sweet Potato				
Potato				
Cereal				
Rice				
Spaghetti, Noodles, Macaroni				
Bread				

Adherence Tool 9–1 continued

Biscuits, Rolls				
Crackers				
Potato chips				
Doughnuts				
Cake, Cookies				
Pie, Pastry				
Sugar				
Syrup, Honey				
Candy				
Jelly, Jam				
Salt				
Coffee				
Decaffeinated Coffee				
Tea				
Soft Drinks				
Beer, Wine				
Whiskey				
Frozen TV Dinners				
Commercial Soup				
Pepper				
Chili Powder				
Cocoa				

What drug products are you taking currently?_____
Who does the food shopping?_____
Where do you eat most of your meals?_____

Adherence Tool 9–2 Informational Device

Goal Chart for a Bland Diet

My goal is to alter my eating behavior by including ___meals per day. The volume of each meal will be reduced by ___the usual intake. I will accomplish this on a daily basis.

√ = I did not decrease
the volume of each meal by ___.

− = I did not include ___ meals today.

* = I did decrease the volume of
each meal by ___.

** = I did have ___ meals today.

M	Tu	W	Th	F	Sa	Su

2. List three treatment strategies to combat inappropriate eating behaviors in clients on a bland regimen.

   a. _____

   _____

   b. _____

   _____

   c. _____

   _____

3. Mrs. J., who is 30 years old, has just been told by her physician that she must follow a bland diet. In the assessment phase of your counseling you learn that she has a very hectic schedule and feels she will have difficulty working in frequent meals. Identify a strategy you might use to solve the problem and provide a reason for selecting the strategy.

   _____

   _____

   _____

   _____

   _____

   _____

   _____

   _____

4. Identify three questions the client might address in determining whether or not dietary habits are changing so that it is easier to follow a bland regimen.

   a. _____

   _____

   b. _____

   _____

   c. _____

   _____

5. List three questions that might be used in evaluating the nutrition counselor's progress.

   a. _____

   _____

   b. _____

   _____

   c. _____

   _____

NOTES

1. Marie V. Krause and L. Kathleen Mahan, *Food, Nutrition and Diet Therapy* (Philadelphia: W.B. Saunders Company, 1979), 476.

2. American Dietetic Association, *Handbook of Clinical Dietetics* (New Haven, Conn.: Yale University Press, 1981), B23–B28.

3. Camilla Kotrba and Charles F. Code, "Gastric Acid Secretory Response to Some Purified Foods and to Addition of Sucrose or Olive Oil," *American Journal of Digestive Diseases* 14 (1969): 1.

4. James P. Koch and Robert M. Donaldson, "A Survey of Food Intolerances in Hospitalized Patients," *New England Journal of Medicine* 271 (1964): 657.

5. J.E. Lennard-Jones and N. Barbouris, "Effect of Different Foods on the Acidity of the Gastric Contents in Patients with Duodenal Ulcer. Part I. A Comparison between Two 'Therapeutic' Diets and Freely Chosen Meals," *Gut* 6 (1965): 113.

SUGGESTED READINGS

Books

Ingelfinger, Franz J., ed. *Controversy in Internal Medicine II.* Philadelphia: W.B. Saunders Company, 1974.

Krause, Marie V., and Mahan, L. Kathleen. *Food, Nutrition and Diet Therapy.* Philadelphia: W.B. Saunders Company, 1979.

Mitchell, Helen S. *Nutrition in Health and Disease.* Philadelphia: J.B. Lippincott Co., 1976.

Rubin, H. *The Ulcer Diet Cookbook.* New York: M. Evans and Company, 1963.

Sleisenger, Marvin H., and Fordtram, John S., eds. *Gastrointestinal Disease,* 2nd rev. ed. Philadelphia: W.B. Saunders Company, 1978.

Spiro, Howard M. *Clinical Gastroenterology,* 2nd rev. ed. New York: Macmillan Publishing Co., 1977.

Thorn, George W. *Harrison's Principles of Internal Medicine,* 8th rev. ed. New York: McGraw Hill Book Company, 1977.

Articles

Boden, Guenther. "Effect of Nicotine on Serum Secretin and Exocrine Pancreatic Secretion." *American Journal of Digestive Diseases* 21(1976):974–977.

Brown, Malcolm. "Personality Factors in Duodenal Ulcer Disease." *Psychosomatic Medicine* 12(1950):1–5.

Brunner, Lillian S. "What to Do (and What to Teach Your Patient) About Peptic Ulcer." *Nursing '76* 6(1976):27–34.

Buchman, Elwood; Kaung, David T; and Knapp, Ruth N. "Dietary Treatment in Duodenal Ulcer." *American Journal of Clinical Nutrition* 22(1969):1536–1542.

———. "Unrestricted Diet in the Treatment of Duodenal Ulcer." *Gastroenterology* 56(1969):1016–1020.

Cohen, Sidney, and Booth, Glenn H., Jr. "Gastric Acid Secretion and Lower Esophageal Sphincter Pressure in Response to Coffee and Caffeine." *New Engand Journal of Medicine* 293(1975):897–899.

Demling, L., and Koch, H. "Condiments." *Acta Hepato-Gastroenterology* 21(1974):377.

Doll, R.; Friedlander, Peter; and Pygott, Frank. "Dietetic Treatment of Peptic Ulcer." *Lancet* 1(1956):5–9.

Donaldson, Robert M., Jr. "The Muddle of Diets for Gastrointestinal Disorders." *Journal of the American Medical Association* 225(1973):1243.

Friedman, Gary S.; Siegelaub, A.B.; and Seltzer, Carl C. "Cigarettes, Alcohol, Coffee and Peptic Ulcer." *New England Journal of Medicine* 290(1974):469–473.

Gillespie, Iain E. "Disease of the Digestive System. Duodenal Ulcer." *British Medical Journal* 4(1967):281–284.

Groisser, Daniel S. "A Study of Caffeine in Tea. I. A New Spectophotometric Micro Method. II. Concentration of Caffeine in Various Strengths, Brands, Blends and Types of Teas." *American Journal of Clinical Nutrition* 31(1978):1727–1731.

Grossman, Morton I. "A New Look at Peptic Ulcer." *Annals of Internal Medicine* 84(1976):57–67.

Hunt, D.R., and Forrest, A.P.M. "The Role of the Antrum in Determining the Acid Secretory Response to Meals of Different Consistency." *Gut* 16(1975):774–776.

Ippoliti, Andrew F.; Maxwell, Vernon; and Isenberg, Jon I. "The Effect of Various Forms of Milk on Gastric Acid Secretion, Studies in Patients with Duodenal Ulcer and Normal Subjects." *Annals of Internal Medicine* 84(1976):286–289.

Isenberg, Jon I. "Peptic Ulcer Disease." *Postgraduate Medicine* 57(1975):163–168.

———. "Therapy of Peptic Ulcer." *Journal of the American Medical Association* 233(1975):540–542.

Kirsner, Joseph B. "Facts and Fallacies of Current Medical Therapy for Uncomplicated Duodenal Ulcer." *Journal of the American Medical Association* 187(1964):423–428.

Kramer, Philip, and Caso, Elizabeth K. "Is the Rationale for Gastrointestinal Diet Therapy Sound?" *Journal of the American Dietetic Association* 42(1963):505–510.

Lennard-Jones, J.E., and Barbouris, N. "Effect of Different Foods on the Acidity of the Gastric Contents in Patients with Duodenal Ulcer. Part I. A Comparison Between Two 'Therapeutic' Diets and Freely Chosen Meals." *Gut* 6(1965):113–117.

McKegney, F. Patrick. "Psychosomatic Aspects of Gastrointestinal Disease." *Postgraduate Medicine* 57(1975):43–47.

Odell, Amy C. "Ulcer Dietotherapy: Past and Present." *Journal of the American Dietetic Association* 58(1971):447–450.

Piper, Douglas W. "Milk in the Treatment of Gastric Disease." *American Journal of Clinical Nutrition* 22(1969):191–195.

Roth, Harold P., and Caron, Herbert S. "Patients' Misconceptions About Their Peptic Ulcer Diets: Potential Obstacles to Cooperation." *Journal of Chronic Diseases* 20(1967):5–11.

Shull, Harrison J. "Diet in the Management of Peptic Ulcer." *Journal of the American Medical Association* 170(1959):1068–1071.

Snorf, Lowell D. "Emotional Factors in Gastrointestinal Disorders." *Journal of the American Medical Association* 162(1956):857–860.

Solanke, Toriola F. "The Effect of Red Pepper (capsicum frutescens) on Gastric Acid Secretion." *Journal of Surgical Research* 15(1973):385–390.

Todd, John W. "Treatment of Peptic Ulcer." *Lancet* 1(1952):113–118.

Weinstein, Louis. "Diet as Related to Gastrointestinal Function." *Journal of the American Medical Association* 176(1961):935–941.

Williams, C.B.; Forrest, A.P., and Campbell, H. "Buffering Capacity of Food in Relation to Stimulation of Gastric Secretion." *Gastroenterology* 55(1968):567–574.

Chapter 10

Termination and Follow-Up

Objectives for Chapter 10

1. Identify strategies to assure dietary adherence after ceasing reinforcement.
2. Generate the reinstitution of an intervention or treatment plan.

10

STRATEGIES TO ASSURE ADHERENCE

When counseling on nutrition-related issues, follow-up interviewing sessions are extremely important. The number of clients' return visits will depend on the success of their efforts in following a diet. There will always be a point at which the nutrition practitioners and clients must end a set of counseling sessions. This is the point at which counselors must be sure that the clients can follow the diet without continued help. At that time, the true goal of the counseling session is tested: Can the clients function alone in the real world?

Counselors must be sure that their clients are given ample opportunity during the sessions to practice eating behaviors and be reinforced for them in the natural environment. This can be done by asking them for records of foods consumed, times eating takes place, persons present during the meal or snack, and the type of situation (where and what type of function). These records should be discussed thoroughly with the clients and problem areas and their solutions noted.

To help with reinforcement in the natural setting, the clients are asked to list times and places where their eating behaviors can be supported. The counselors then help them plan for natural environmental situations that will reinforce the new eating pattern. If new behaviors are really adjustive, they should find natural support and natural reinforcements.

In early stages of termination, the counselors should help the clients identify chains of events that bolster behavior. A woman who had succeeded in losing 10 pounds found that her colleagues at work responded very warmly to her. She was asked out more often and spent more time in discussions with colleagues. She eliminated her clothes-buying reinforcement and instead posted a sign on her refrigerator door: "Dieting keeps the telephone ringing!"

After an eating behavior has been solidified in relation to one antecedent condition, clients can make that behavior even more frequent by gradually increasing the range of situations in which reinforcement occurs. They should test for generalization by looking at how reinforcement can be a part of many situations. By keeping a list of all situations in which either appropriate or inappropriate eating behaviors occur, nutritionists can work on problem situations before counseling is terminated.

A most important issue to address before termination is building in resistance to extinction. The best way to assure that an appropriate eating behavior continues is to work out an intermittent reinforcement schedule. A treatment plan never should be stopped abruptly.

Once an acceptable upper level of behavior has been established, the ratio of its reinforcement can be reduced. Instead of the clients' always buying presents for themselves, such as clothing, after eating an appropriate meal, sporadic buying can be used as a reinforcement, i.e., 75 percent of the time, then 50 percent, then 25 percent, and so on.

It is important to keep in mind that during this gradual reduction in positive reinforcement, both counselors and clients must continue to count the frequency of the appropriate behaviors. There is some danger that these will decline. Alternating between periods of 50 percent and 100 percent reinforcement can keep their frequency at an acceptably high level if the natural supporters are slow to evolve.

Counselors should ensure that adequate practice of the reinforcement has occurred during intervention or treatment. In general, acceptable behaviors are made more probable by providing a certain number of trials on a reinforcement schedule. Practice is important.

This need for practice implies, correctly, that nutrition counselors will not want to terminate the program as soon as the goal is reached. Instead, it would be wise to continue the plan for a week or two, or perhaps more, depending on the frequency of opportunities to practice. The number of practices depends on many factors in the intervention plan.

However, a trial at reducing reinforcement is a good test of the degree to which an eating behavior can be maintained after termination. If the frequency of the targeted behavior drops alarmingly as soon as a reduction in reinforcement begins, it means more practice is necessary. In that case, the 100 percent reinforcement schedule should be resumed, along with more practice. For this reason, the frequency of an eating behavior should be recorded after termination of reinforcement until the rate has stabilized.

REINSTITUTION OF INTERVENTION OR TREATMENT

Nutrition counselors may find that an intervention plan must be restarted if gradually decreasing reinforcement seems to be causing an appropriate eating behavior to drop off. At that point, practitioners must be very attuned to client needs.

In some cases, events in clients' lives may be affecting their adherence to the diet. Such events can involve many of the following problems that psychologists believe cause major changes in life styles:

1. death in family
2. illness in family
3. client's illness
4. loss of job
5. new job
6. retirement
7. moving (relocating)
8. financial difficulties
9. divorce/separation
10. children leaving home
11. birth of a child

Because clients must deal with other problems, their attention to an intervention strategy of gradually decreasing reinforcement may have been diverted, resulting in total lack of support.

By working with clients' significant others, practitioners can provide people who will reinforce good eating behaviors in the absence of nutrition counseling sessions.

THE TERMINATION PROCESS

The algorithm in Figure 10–1 indicates a step procedure to use in terminating nutrition counseling. Termination always should be approached gradually. Some clients will respond well to this, others may have problems. The algorithm indicates four possible situations:

1. This involves clients who begin having negative thoughts. The algorithm suggests listing those thoughts and working on them.
2. Clients occasionally may refuse to discuss them, in which case they should be asked to record both negative and positive monologues for discussion later.
3. Other clients may admit to having a drastic change in their life styles. Those changes may be temporary. In that case, the intervention plan is reinstituted and reinforcements decreased gradually.
4. Clients in some cases may be in the midst of a change in life style. If so, counselors should wait until they seem ready to restart the

Figure 10–1 Algorithm for Nutrition Counseling Termination

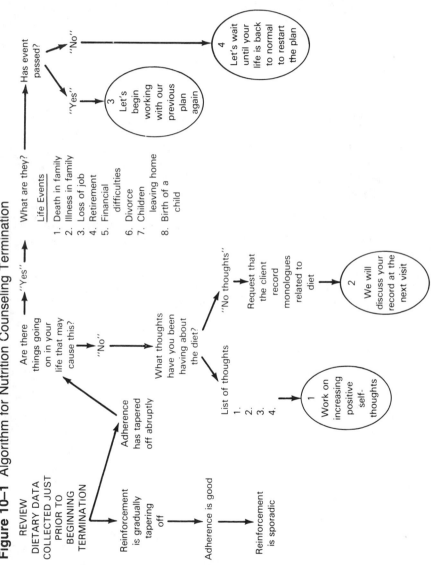

intervention plan, meanwhile keeping in close contact so that the diet is not totally forgotten.

Termination will be different for each client. Counselors should be prepared to restart a strategy to help assure adherence to the diet over long periods. They also should call or write clients periodically to check on their progress. Such attention to the clients' needs after the counseling has ended will show that the dietitians or nutritionists care and may help maintain the individuals' motivation.

A gradual fading process of termination rather than an abrupt "goodbye" is essential. If clients are to be successful on their own, they must prove that success is possible. Nutrition counselors can help clients find this success on their own. Absence of a gradual termination can prove frustrating to clients at being abruptly left on their own and may send them back to their problem behaviors.

REVIEW OF CHAPTER 10
(Answers in Appendix I)

1. Identify five ways in which you as a counselor might facilitate the continuation of appropriate dietary behaviors in clients who no longer will be coming in for interviews and must live with the regimen in the real world.
   a. _____
   b. _____
   c. _____
   d. _____
   e. _____
2. Mr Y. has been slipping in his adherence to the low-sodium regimen he was following so well when counseling sessions were frequent. What questions might you use to determine exactly what has happened to the reinforcement schedule?_____
   _____
   _____
   _____

3. What intervention plan can you recommend to help clients maintain dietary adherence?_____
   _____
   _____
   _____

SUGGESTED READINGS

Books

Aronson, Virginia, and Fitzgerald, Barbara D. *Guidebook for Nutrition Counselors.* North Quincy, Mass.: The Christopher Publishing House, 1980.

Cormier, William H., and Cormier, L. Sherilyn. *Interviewing Strategies for Helpers: A Guide to Assessment, Treatment and Evaluation.* Monterey, Calif.: Brooks/Cole Publishing Company, 1979.

Eisenberg, S., and Delaney, D.J. *The Counseling Process*, 2nd rev. ed. Chicago: Rand McNally Publishing Company, 1977.

Hackney, H., and Cormier, L. Sherilyn. *Counseling Strategies and Objectives*, 2nd rev. ed. Englewood Cliffs, N.J.: Prentice-Hall, 1979.

Pietrofesa, John J.; *Counseling: Theory, Research, and Practice.* Chicago: Rand McNally Publishing Company, 1978.

Stewart, Norman R. *Systematic Counseling.* Englewood Cliffs, N.J.: Prentice-Hall, 1978.

Watson, David L., and Tharp, Roland G. *Self-Directed Behavior: Self-Modification for Personal Adjustment.* Monterey, Calif.: Brooks/Cole Publishing Company, 1972.

Glossary

Adherence: Maintenance of a schedule over a selected period of time.

Adherence Tool: Written information and/or verbal instructions that help clients reach targeted goals.

Baseline Data: Information collected about clients that describes their situation before beginning an intervention, such as weight-control or low-sodium eating patterns, etc.

Behavioral Therapy: A counseling treatment practice that involves a combination of all principles of learning. Its strength lies in its combination of action and fantasy techniques. Behavioral treatment professionals generally are expert in the analysis of chains of events, in the arrangement of antecedents, and in the design and management of contingencies. When individuals cannot manage to control their natural environment, therapists may begin imaginative assertive training in which the clients imagine a situation and counselors verbally guide the fantasy.

Client: Person with whom a nutrition counselor is working to formulate a change in eating behaviors.

Client-Centered Therapy: A counseling technique that involves regular, private conversations between counselors and clients. The counselors create a special environment by using a noncritical, accepting attitude toward whatever the clients say. Counselors must signal by speech or gesture their acceptance of a very broad range of statements about thoughts and feelings. The counselors' comments are limited primarily to brief questions or restatements of client statements, especially those about feelings, in order to clarify exactly what the individuals mean. This extremely simple technique can be more difficult to manage than it sounds. It is very powerful.

Coaching Aids: Instructions about the general principles for performing a desired behavior effectively.

Cognitive Restructuring: A process in which clients learn to turn negative thoughts into positive ones.

Contracting: The counselors' act of forming an agreement with clients to perform a specific behavior, a certain number of times, in a certain way, within a given time period. The contract may have a built-in reward for achieving the specified behavior.

Coping: An indication of strength through a behavior that is creative, constructive, or responsible.

Counseling: A mutual process by counselors and clients in which the latter learn new behaviors and thought processes that help with decision-making skills and problem resolution.

Covert Process: A private process, e.g., an internal activity, not directly observable to someone else, such as clients' thoughts, beliefs, emotions, and feelings.

Cues: A variety of stimuli to help promote or extinguish a behavior.

Dietary Behavior: Observable acts involved in habitual eating-related events in clients' daily lives.

Eating Behavior: See dietary behavior.

Environmental Stimuli: Objects, events, persons in the clients' world that cue or stimulate eating behaviors.

Extinction: Elimination of a behavior.

Food Behavior: See dietary behavior.

Gestalt Therapy: A counseling process that emphasizes the "now." The past is a memory, the future is a fantasy, and both are important only as they are experienced in the present. Nonverbal behavior is very important in Gestalt therapy.

Induction Aids: Supportive aids arranged by counselors to assist clients in performing difficult behaviors.

Kinetics: Body motion, i.e., gestures, body movements, facial expressions, eye behavior, and posture.

Learning Games: Simulations of actual events to help clients deal with problem behaviors in actual situations.

Modeling: A procedure by which clients can learn through observing and mimicking the behavior of others.

- **Mastery Modeling:** Modeling an ideal situation, as things should be.
- **Coping Modeling:** Modeling in which errors in performance may be evidenced.

Nutrition Counseling: A relationship between a professionally trained, competent nutritionist/dietitian and an individual seeking help in following a special diet. The nutrition counselor helps the client gain knowledge about the diet, greater self-understanding, and improved decision-making and behavior-change skills for problem resolution.

Nutrition Practitioners: Dietitians or nutritionists who deal with nutrition problems in free-living clients.

Overt: Any visible activity that clients perform or demonstrate.

Paralinguistics: Voice qualities and vocalizations, i.e., voice level, pitch and fluency of speech.

Proxemics: The use of social and personal space, i.e., size of the room, seating arrangements, and distance between counselors and clients.

Rational Emotive Therapy: A counseling process in which the main purposes are (1) to demonstrate to clients that negative self-talk is the source of disturbance and (2) to re-evaluate this negative self-talk in order to eliminate it and its resulting illogical ideas.

Reinforcement: A reward for a behavior.

- **Positive Reinforcement:** A reward for a behavior that consists of a pleasant consequence.
- **Negative Reinforcement:** A reward that consists of a punishing or unpleasant consequence for not exhibiting the behavior.

Responses: Verbal or nonverbal acts or thoughts in reaction to verbal or nonverbal stimuli.

Satiation: Fullness, satisfaction.

Sequenced Learning: Acquisition of knowledge and or skills in a step-by-step fashion.

Situational Cues: Encouragement of a behavior by associating it with an event in the clients' environment.

Situational Variables: Changing events in clients' environment.

Staging: The process of introducing information or change gradually. Small steps in providing information or making changes make major goals realizable.

Stimuli: Environmental conditions that serve as cues for or antecedents of a particular response.

Strategy: A plan for attainment of a specified goal.

Tailoring: A means of gearing information or behavior change to clients' life styles.

Thought Stopping: A process for helping clients control unproductive or self-defeating thoughts by suppressing or eliminating them.

Verbal Setting Operation: An activity that attempts to predispose someone to view a situation or an event in a certain way before that event actually takes place.

Checklist of Counselor Self-Image

Check the items that are most descriptive of you.

1. *Competence Assessment*

_____ 1. Constructive negative feedback about myself doesn't make me feel incompetent or uncertain of myself.

_____ 2. I tend to put myself down frequently.

_____ 3. I feel fairly confident about myself as a helper.

_____ 4. I often am preoccupied with thinking that I'm not going to be a competent nutrition counselor.

_____ 5. When I am involved in a conflict, I don't go out of my way to ignore or avoid it.

_____ 6. When I get positive feedback about myself, I often don't believe it's true.

_____ 7. I set realistic goals for myself as a helper that are within reach.

_____ 8. I believe that a confronting, hostile client could make me feel uneasy or incompetent.

_____ 9. I often find myself apologizing for myself or my behavior.

_____ 10. I'm fairly confident I can or will be a successful counselor.

_____ 11. I find myself worrying a lot about "not making it" as a counselor.

_____ 12. I'm likely to be a little scared by clients who would idealize me.

_____ 13. A lot of times I will set standards or goals for myself that are too tough to attain.

_____ 14. I tend to avoid negative feedback when I can.

_____ 15. Doing well or being successful does not make me feel uneasy.

Source: Reprinted from *Interviewing Strategies for Helpers* by William H. Cormier and L. Sherilyn Cormier with permission of Brooks/Cole Publishing Company, © 1979, pp. 14–15.

2. *Power Assessment*

____ 1. If I'm really honest, I think my counseling methods are a little superior to other people's.

____ 2. A lot of times I try to get people to do what I want. I might get pretty defensive or upset if the client disagreed with what I wanted to do or did not follow my direction in the interview.

____ 3. I believe there is (or will be) a balance in the interviews between my participation and the client's.

____ 4. I could feel angry when working with a resistant or stubborn client.

____ 5. I can see that I might be tempted to get some of my own ideology across to the client.

____ 6. As a counselor, "preaching" is not likely to be a problem for me.

____ 7. Sometimes I feel impatient with clients who have a different way of looking at the world than I do.

____ 8. I know there are times when I would be reluctant to refer my clients to someone else, especially if the other counselor's style differed from mine.

____ 9. Sometimes I feel rejecting or intolerant of clients whose values and life styles are very different from mine.

____ 10. It is hard for me to avoid getting in a power struggle with some clients.

3. *Intimacy Assessment*

____ 1. There are times when I act more gruff than I really feel.

____ 2. It's hard for me to express positive feelings to a client.

____ 3. There are some clients I would really like to be my friends more than my clients.

____ 4. It would upset me if a client didn't like me.

____ 5. If I sense a client has some negative feelings toward me, I try to talk about it rather than avoid it.

____ 6. Many times I go out of my way to avoid offending clients.

____ 7. I feel more comfortable maintaining a professional distance between myself and the client.

____ 8. Being close to people is something that does not make me feel uncomfortable.

____ 9. I am more comfortable when I am a little aloof.

____ 10. I am very sensitive to how clients feel about me, especially if it is negative.

____ 11. I can accept positive feedback from clients fairly easily.

____ 12. It is difficult for me to confront a client.

Learning Activity Reaction:
Applications to Your Counseling

1. For each of the three assessment areas above you can look over your responses and determine the areas that seem to be OK and the areas that may be a problem for you or something to watch out for. You may find more problems in one area than another.
2. Do your "trouble spots" seem to occur with mostly everyone, or just with certain types of people? In all situations or some situations?
3. Compare yourself now to where you might have been four years ago or where you may be four years from now.
4. Identify any areas you feel you could use some help with, from a colleague, a supervisor, or a counselor.

Checklist of Nutrition Counselor's Nonverbal Behavior

Instructions: Determine whether the counselor did or did not demonstrate the desired nonverbal behaviors listed in the right column. Check "yes" or "no" in the left column to indicate your judgment.

Demonstrated Behaviors		*Desired Behaviors*
Yes	*No*	
____	____	*Eye contact*—Maintained persistent eye contact
1. Eyes		without gazing or staring.
____	____	*Facial expression*—Punctuated interaction with
2. Head nods		occasional head nods.
____	____	*Mouth*—Punctuated interaction with occasional smiles.
3. Smiles		
____	____	*Body orientation and posture*—Faced the other
4. Facing client		person, slight lean forward (from waist up),
____	____	body appeared relaxed.
5. Leaning forward		
____	____	
6. Relaxed body		

___

____   ____   *Paralinguistics*—Completed sentences without
    7. Completed   "uhs" or hesitations in delivery, asked one
      sentences   question at a time, did not ramble.

____   ____
8. Smooth delivery—
    no speech errors

____   ____   *Distance*—Seats of counselor and client were
9. Distance   between 3 feet, or 1 meter, and 5 feet, or 1½
                                  meters apart.

COMMENTS:

Client Eating Questionnaire

The following questionnaire has been designed to efficiently collect patient information in clinical weight control programs. It has several functions.

Initially, it is a useful screening device or test of motivation. Individuals who will not take time to fill it out probably will not take time to participate fully in the behavioral weight control program.

Secondly, the answers to these questions can be of great use to the therapist during the initial interviews and later during the weight control lessons. The weight history allows him to systematically look at the patients' own views of their weight problems, and at some of the environmental influences they feel are important to their weight problems. The history of past attempts to lose weight, the lengths of time they have stayed in weight loss programs, and the reasons for past failure can all be useful during the 20 weeks of this program. Also, their report of mood changes during previous periods of weight loss can help you anticipate and deal with problems that might arise during treatment.

A brief medical history is included to give you a basis for referral. For example, if someone indicates he or she is a diabetic, and does not have a physician, you might suggest contacting a doctor before the weight control program begins. Similarly, if someone indicates a history of heart disease, you may want to check with that person's physician before dealing with increased activity and exercise.

Source: Adapted from *Learning to Eat, Behavior Modification for Weight Control* by James M. Ferguson with permission of Bull Publishing Co., © 1975, Appendix.

The questions about social and family history provide additional information that is of use medically: for example, the cause of parental death and the family weight history.

In most states the information contained in this questionnaire is confidential. Without *written* approval from the patients, this information cannot be divulged to interested individuals, physicians, insurance companies, or law enforcement agencies.

Name:_____ Sex: M F Age:___ Birthdate:_____

Address:_____ Home phone:_____

_____ Office phone:_____

WEIGHT HISTORY:

1. Your present weight _____ Height _____

2. Describe your present weight (circle one)

       very   slightly   about
   overweight   overweight   average

3. Are you dissatisfied with the way you look at this weight? (circle one)

   Completely   Very
   Satisfied   Satisfied   Neutral   Dissatisfied   Dissatisfied

4. At what weight have you *felt* your best or do you think you would feel your best?

   _____

5. How much weight would you like to lose? _____

6. Do you feel your weight affects your daily activities?

   No effect   Some effect   Often interferes   Extreme effect

7. Why do you want to lose weight at this time? _____

   _____

8. What are the attitudes of the following people about your attempt(s) to lose weight?

	Negative (They disap- prove or are re- sentful)	*Indifferent* (They don't care or don't help)	*Positive* (They encour- age me and are understanding)
Husband			
Wife			
Children			
Parents			
Employer			
Friends			

9. Do these attitudes affect your weight loss or gain?   Yes   No
   If yes, please describe:_____
   _____
   _____

10. Indicate on the following table the periods in your life when you
    have been overweight. *Where appropriate,* list your maximum weight
    for each period and number of pounds you were overweight. Briefly
    describe any methods you used to lose weight in that five-year pe-
    riod, e.g., diet, shots, pills. Also list any significant life events you
    feel were related to either your weight gain or loss, e.g., college
    tests, marriage, pregnancies, illness.

Age	Maximum Weight	Pounds Overweight	Methods Used To Lose Weight	Significant Events Related to Weight Change
Birth				
0 – 5				
5 – 10				
10 – 15				

Age	Maximum Weight	Pounds Overweight	Methods Used To Lose Weight	Significant Events Related to Weight Change
15 – 20				
20 – 25				
25 – 30				
30 – 35				
35 – 40				
40 – 45				
45 – 50				
50 – 55				
55 – 60				
60 – 65				

11. How *physically* active are you? (circle one)

Very active   Active   Average   Inactive   Very inactive

12. What do you do for physical exercise and how often do you do it?

ACTIVITY (for example, swimming, jogging, dancing)	FREQUENCY (daily, weekly, monthly)

13. A number of different ways of losing weight are listed below. Please indicate which methods you have used by filling the appropriate blanks.

	Ages Used	Number of Times Used	Maximum Weight Lost	Comments: Length of Time Weight Loss Maintained; Success; Difficulties
TOPS (Take Off Pounds Sensibly)				
Weight Watchers				
Pills				
Supervised Diet				
Unsupervised Diet				
Starvation				
Behavior Modification				
Psychotherapy				
Hypnosis				
Other				

14. Which method did you use for the longest period of time? _____

_____

15. Have you had a major mood change during or after a significant weight loss? Indicate any mood changes on the following checklist.

	Not at all	A little bit	Moder- ately	Quite a bit	Extremely
a. Depressed, sad, feeling down, un- happy, the blues.	____	____	____	____	____
b. Anxious, nervous, restless, or uptight all the time.	____	____	____	____	____
c. Physically weak.	____	____	____	____	____
d. Elated or happy.	____	____	____	____	____
e. Easily irritated, an- noyed, or angry.	____	____	____	____	____
f. Fatigued, worn out, tired all the time.	____	____	____	____	____
g. A lack of self-confi- dence.	____	____	____	____	____

16. What usually goes wrong with your weight loss programs? _____

_____

_____

_____

MEDICAL HISTORY:

17. When did you last have a complete physical examination? _____

18. Who is your current doctor? _____

19. What medical problems do you have at the present time? _____

_____

_____

20. What medications or drugs do you take regularly? _____

_____

_____

21. List any medications, drugs or foods you are allergic to _____

_____

_____

22. List any hospitalizations or operations. Indicate how old you were at each hospital admission.

    Age   Reason for hospitalizations

    _____   _____

    _____   _____

23. List any serious illnesses you have had which have not required hospitalization. Indicate how old you were during each illness.

    Age   Illness

    _____   _____

    _____   _____

    _____   _____

    _____   _____

24. Describe any of your medical problems that are complicated by excess weight.

_____

_____

_____

_____

_____

25. How much alcohol do you usually drink per week? _____

26. List any psychiatric contact, individual counseling, or marital counseling that you have had or are now having.

    Age   Reason for contact and type of therapy

    _____   _____

    _____   _____

    _____   _____

    _____   _____

SOCIAL HISTORY:

27. Circle the last year of school attended:

    1 2 3 4 5 6 7 8   9 10 11 12   1 2 3 4   M.A.   Ph.D.
       Grade School   High School   College

    Other _____

28. Describe your present occupation _____

    _____

29. How long have you worked for your present employer? _____

30. Present marital status (circle one):

    single   married   divorced   widowed   separated   engaged

31. Answer the following questions for each marriage:

    Dates of marriages   _____   _____   _____
    Date of termination   _____   _____   _____
    Reason (death, divorce, etc.) _____   _____   _____
    Number of children   _____   _____   _____

32. Spouse's Age _____ Weight _____ Height _____

33. Describe your spouse's occupation _____

    _____

34. Describe your spouse's weight   (circle one)

    very   slightly   about   slightly   very
    overweight   overweight   average   underweight underweight

35. List your children's ages, sex, heights, weights, and circle whether
    they are overweight, average, or underweight. Include any children
    from previous marriages, whether they are living with you or not.

    Age Sex Weight Height   Overweight   Underweight

    ____ ___ _____ _____ very   slightly   average   slightly   very
    ____ ___ _____ _____ very   slightly   average   slightly   very
    ____ ___ _____ _____ very   slightly   average   slightly   very
    ____ ___ _____ _____ very   slightly   average   slightly   very
    ____ ___ _____ _____ very   slightly   average   slightly   very

36. Who lives at home with you? _____

FAMILY HISTORY:

37. Is your father living?   Yes   No   Father's age now, or age at and cause of death _____

_____

38. Is your mother living?   Yes   No   Mother's age now, or age at and cause of death _____

_____

39. Describe your father's occupation _____

40. Describe your mother's occupation _____

41. Describe your father's weight while you were growing up (circle one).

    very   slightly   about   slightly   very
    overweight   overweight   average   underweight   underweight

42. Describe your mother's weight while you were growing up (circle one).

    very   slightly   about   slightly   very
    overweight   overweight   average   underweight   underweight

43. List your brothers' and sisters' ages, sex, present weights, heights, and circle whether they are overweight, average, or underweight.

Age	Sex	Weight	Height	Overweight			Underweight	
____	____	_____	_____	very	slightly	average	slightly	very
____	____	_____	_____	very	slightly	average	slightly	very
____	____	_____	_____	very	slightly	average	slightly	very
____	____	_____	_____	very	slightly	average	slightly	very
____	____	_____	_____	very	slightly	average	slightly	very

44. Please add any additional information you feel may be relevant to your weight problem. This includes interactions with your family and friends that might sabotage a weight-loss program, and addi-

tional family or social history that you feel might help us understand
your weight problem.

_____

_____

_____

_____

_____

_____

_____

_____

Behavioral Chart

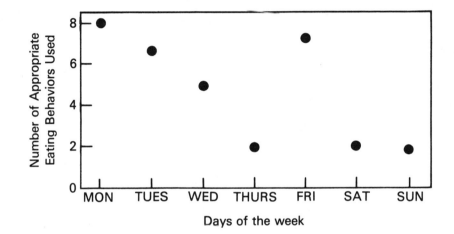

Days of the week

Behavioral Log

Date	Time	Setting	Event	Actual Reaction	Desired Reaction

Logs of Thoughts Related to Food

Baseline Log

Time	Thoughts
7:30	"I'd really like a doughnut but I'm not going to blow my day."
8:15	"It's not fair, I'm really trying and I haven't lost anything."
9:10	"Wish I had a doughnut or something. I'm hungry."
10:00	"It's not fair, it's snack time and all I get is water."
11:30	"Nothing tastes as good when I know there's no dessert."
12:10	"Look at them. They stuff themselves with sweets and stay skinny."
1:15	"Maybe I could have just a couple of cookies after school. I've earned them."
2:30	"Look at them running off to their afternoon snacks. It's not fair."
3:15	"I don't care if I'm fat. I'll never lose anyway. It's not worth it."
4:30	"I might as well eat and enjoy it. I'll never lose anyway. It's not worth it."
5:45	"You pig. Now you feel stuffed and you've ruined your day."
7:30	"What a failure I am. I don't deserve to be thin."
9:00	"I'll never learn, will I? It's no use."
10:30	"I feel hopeless. I've tried everything and I always blow it."

Source: Reprinted from *Permanent Weight Control, A Total Solution to the Dieter's Dilemma* by Michael J. Mahoney and Kathryn Mahoney with permission of W. W. Norton & Company, Inc., © 1976, pp. 65, 62–63.

Replacement Log

Problem Category	Negative Monologues	Appropriate Monologues
Pounds Lost	"I'm not losing fast enough." "I've starved myself and haven't lost a thing." "I've been more consistent than Mary and she is losing faster than I am. It's not fair."	"Pounds don't count. If I continue my eating habits, the pounds will be lost." "Have patience—those pounds took a long time to get there. As long as they stay off permanently, I'll settle for any progress." "It takes a while to break down fat and absorb the extra water produced. I'm not going to worry about it."
Capabilities	"I just don't have the willpower." "I'm just naturally fat." "Why should this work—nothing else has." "I'll probably just regain it." "What the heck—I'd rather be fat than miserable. Besides, I'm not that heavy."	"There's no such thing as lack of willpower—just poor planning." "If I make a few improvements here and there and take things one day at a time, I can be very successful." "It's going to be nice to be permanently rid of all this extra baggage. I'm starting to feel better already."
Excuses	"If it weren't for my job and the kids, I could lose weight." "It's just impossible to eat right with a schedule like mine." "I'm just so nervous all the time—I have to eat to satisfy my psychological needs." "Maybe next time. . . ."	"My schedule isn't any worse than anyone else's. What I need to do is be a bit more creative in how to improve my eating." "Eating doesn't satisfy psychological problems—it creates them." "Job, kids, or whatever, I'm the one in control."

Replacement Log continued

Goals	"Well, there goes my diet. That coffee cake probably cost me two pounds, and after I promised myself—no more sweets." "I always blow it on the weekends." "Fine—I start the day off with a doughnut. I may as well enjoy myself today."	"What is this—the Olympics? I don't need perfect habits, just improved ones." "Why should one sweet or an extra portion blow it for me? I'll cut back elsewhere." "Those high standards are unrealistic." "Fantastic—I had a small piece of cake and it didn't blow the day."
Food Thoughts	"I can't stop thinking about sweets." "I had images of cakes and pies all afternoon—it must mean that I need sugar." "When we order food at a restaurant, I continue thinking about what I have ordered until it arrives."	"Whenever I find myself thinking about food, I quickly change the topic to some other pleasant experience." "If I see a magazine ad or commercial for food and I start thinking about it, I distract my attention by doing something else (phoning a friend, getting the mail, etc.)."

Daily Record of Cognitive Restructuring

Date: _____		Record of: _____	
Description of Situation	Coping Thoughts Used	Positive Self-Statements Used	Date and Time

Source: Adapted from *Interviewing Strategies for Helpers* by William H. Cormier and L. Sherilyn Cormier with permission of Brooks/Cole Publishing Company, © 1979, p. 370.

Food Composition Table*

Food Composition Table

(Fat and Cholesterol Content of Certain Foods)

Product	Unit of Measure	Choles- terol mg.	Total[1] Fat gm.	Sat.[2] Fat gm.	Poly[3] Fat gm.	P/S*
Egg	1 whole	252	5.8	1.70	.69	
LRC Meat Composite[4]	1 oz.	27	3.5	1.37	.27	
Beef						
Lean (10%)	1 oz.	26	2.7	.94	.15	
Med. fat (15%)	1 oz.	26	4.4	1.79	.22	
Pork						
Lean (10%)	1 oz.	25	2.8	.86	.27	
Med. fat (15%)	1 oz.	25	4.0	1.34	.43	

[1,2,3] Total fat and fatty acids from Nutrition Coding Center Information Listing Table, 1977.

[4] Weighting for these figures was done by extrapolation of U.S. meat consumption data for 1976 from National Food Situation, Economic Research Service, U.S.D.A., March 1977. Total consumption from meat group: red meat 70.2 percent, poultry 24.0 percent, fish 5.7 percent.

[5] Average of chicken and turkey fat.

[6] This is gravy without milk, figuring just the amount of added fat from meat or poultry.

[0] Average of chicken and turkey fat.

* P/S is a ratio resulting from dividing the grams of polyunsaturated fat by the saturated fat content of the diet.

* Based on the April 1977 revised figures of the Nutrition Coding Center, Minneapolis, Minn., Food Table Information Listing.

Source: Joan Bickel, Karen Smith, Linda G. Snetselaar, and Laura Vailas.

Product	Unit of Measure	Choles-terol mg.	Total[1] Fat gm.	Sat.[2] Fat gm.	Poly[3] Fat gm.	P/S*
Organ meats & cold cuts						
Luncheon meat						
(Beef bologna)	1 oz.	15	8.5	3.77	.38	
Frankfurter	1 oz.	18	7.7	2.85	.90	
Liver (pork, beef, & calf)	1 oz.	166	1.4	.52	.23	
Liver (chicken)	1 oz.	211	1.2	.47	.27	
Poultry						
With skin[0] (lt. meat)	1 oz.	30	1.5	.42	.39	
(dk. meat)	1 oz.	37	2.4	.67	.63	
Without skin (lt. meat)	1 oz.	22	1.0	.25	.22	
(dk. meat)	1 oz.	27	1.8	.48	.44	
Fish						
Flat (12% fat)	1 oz.	32	5.1	.86	1.72	
Flat (2% fat)	1 oz.	25	.3	.08	.14	
Shellfish (oysters)	1 oz.	13	.6	.21	.24	
Crustaceans (crab & lob-ster)	1 oz.	26	.6	.07	.20	
Shrimp	1 oz.	43	.3	.04	.12	
Milk						
Whole	1 cp.	32	8.4	5.28	.31	
2%	1 cp.	14	4.8	2.88	.19	
Milk (1%)	1 cp.	7	2.4	1.44	.07	
Skim (<1% milk fat)	1 cp.	4	.2	.14	.00	
Chocolate drink (2%)	1 cp.	16	5.5	2.16	.14	
Cream						
Heavy (35% fat)	1 tb.	21	5.6	3.53	.21	
Light, sour (20% fat)	1 tb.	10	3.1	1.92	.12	
Half and half (12% fat)	1 tb.	6	1.8	1.10	.06	
Imitation creamer						
(Liquid, sat. fat)	1 tb.	0	1.7	1.28	.00	
(Liquid, P/S 2.0)		0	1.5	.23	.59	
(Liquid, P/S 1.0–2.0)		0	1.4	.27	.45	
Imitation sour cream	1 tb.	0	2.4	2.21	.01	
Ice cream (10% fat)	½ cp.	27	7.0	4.38	.26	
Ice milk	½ cp.	13	4.5	2.80	.17	
Yogurt (1.7% fat)	1 cp.	17	4.1	2.40	.10	
Cheese						
American (20% fat)	1 oz.	29	9.1	5.68	.34	
Cream (35% fat)	1 tb.	15	5.3	2.97	.17	
Mozzarella (part skim)	1 oz.	19	4.7	2.89	.14	
Cottage cheese (4%)	½ cp.	18	5.1	3.19	.15	
Cheezola (corn oil)	1 oz.	1.2	6.5	.83	3.80	

Product	Unit of Measure	Choles- terol mg.	Total[1] Fat gm.	Sat.[2] Fat gm.	Poly[3] Fat gm.	P/S*
Butter	1 ts.	11	3.8	2.33	.14	
Vegetable oils						
Mayonnaise	1 ts.	4	4.0	.60	2.31	3.9
Miracle Whip	1 ts.	0	2.1	.35	1.11	3.2
Mixed oil						
(90% soy; 10% cotns)	1 ts.	—	4.7	.75	2.66	3.6
Crisco oil	1 ts.	—	5.0	.65	1.95	3.0
Crisco, solid	1 ts.	—	4.0	1.00	1.00	1.0
Mazola oil	1 ts.	—	4.7	.62	2.83	4.6
Margarine						
P/S 2.6–4.0						
Promise soft	1 ts.	—	3.7	.63	2.07	3.22
P/S 1.6–1.9						
Fleischmann stick 5/77	1 ts.	—	3.7	.71	1.21	1.7
P/S 2.0–2.5						
Mazola stick 5/77	1 ts.	—	3.8	.67	1.33	2.0
P/S 2.0–2.5						
Fleischmann soft 5/77	1 ts.	—	3.7	.70	1.57	2.2
Parkay soft 7/77	1 ts.	—	3.76	.73	1.17	1.6
P/S .5–1.0						
Parkay regular 7/77	1 ts.	—	3.8	.73	.32	.45
Blue Bonnet stick 5/77	1 ts.	—	3.8	.77	.52	.7
Peanut butter	1 ts.	—	2.7	.51	.81	1.6
Peanuts	1 cp.	—	70.1	13.39	21.04	1.6
Meat fat						
Gravy, beef	¼ cp.	1	1.7	.76	.07	
poultry[5,6]	¼ cp.	1	1.7	.49	.44	
Bacon fat	1 ts.	3	4.7	1.64	.52	
Bacon	1 sl.	6	3.9	1.36	.41	
Lard	1 ts.	4	4.3	1.71	.51	
Beef fat	1 ts.	4	4.4	2.12	.18	
Baked products	1 sv.	44	10.4	2.80	1.73	
Chocolate	1 oz.	0	10.0	6.22	.30	

Answers to Chapter Reviews

Each answer should be discussed in depth. The responses provided here are intended only as general suggestions to help initiate discussion.

Answers to Review of Chapter 4

1. a. "I'm off that rotten diet now" syndrome.
   b. "I'm such a rotten person, what's the use" syndrome.
2. a. Identify the general problem.
   b. Collect data.
   c. Identify inappropriate eating pattern and possible ways toward improvement.
3. a. Substituting nonfood-related activities.
   b. Interposing time.
   c. Eliminating cues.
   d. Involving spouse, family, and friends.
   e. Thinking positively.
   f. Engaging in physical activity.
4. For the client who has a very negative self-concept, I would use the positive thinking strategy. By substituting positive thoughts for negative, self-concepts may become more positive.
5. a. Was the goal reached?
   b. Were eating patterns changed?
   c. Is food quality improved?
   d. Is food quantity reduced?
   e. Has activity level increased?
   f. Are food-related thoughts more positive?
   g. Has the client eliminated eating cues?

6. a. Was the major problem addressed?
    b. Was the client's goal achieved?
    c. Were strategies to alter behavior efficient?
    d. Did I use appropriate verbal and nonverbal interviewing skills?
    e. Did I use appropriate counseling skills?
    f. What changes would I incorporate into the next interview?

Answers to Review of Chapter 5

1. a. "Any vegetable oil is OK on a fat-modified diet."
    b. "One single food will lower my cholesterol so I really don't need to worry about eating other foods."
    c. "My family makes me eat high-fat crackers."
    d. "I can't get by on only six ounces of meat. It's not healthy."
    e. "That low-fat cheese is terrible!"
    f. "I practically drink vegetable oil because I know it will lower my cholesterol level."
2. a. Cholesterol.
    b. Saturated fat.
    c. Polyunsaturated fat.
3. a. Tailor the diet to take past eating habits into consideration.
    b. Stage the diet instruction.
    c. Clear up misconceptions about fat and cholesterol.

4.

	Cholesterol	Total Fat	Saturated Fat	Polyunsaturated Fat
0 egg/week	0	0	0	0
7 oz. meat/day	189	24.5	9.59	1.89
0 dairy	0	0	0	0
2 tsps. Fleischmann's margarine/day	0	7.4	1.42	3.14
3 tsps. Mazola oil/day	0	14.1	1.86	8.49
		46.0	12.87	13.52
			P/S = 1.04	
(% of 2,400 calories)		(18%)		(5%)

Strategies: Jim might tell his friends how important it is to his health to eat foods low in cholesterol and fat. He also might ask his family to help by positively reinforcing his efforts on social occasions. Using skim milk would provide needed calcium.

5. a. Have dietary patterns changed while remaining compatible with life style?
    b. Have misconceptions been replaced with facts?

   c. Are social occasions fun now?

   d. Do family and friends provide positive reinforcement?

6. a. Does assessment allow for tailoring a dietary pattern?

   b. Does the pattern fit in with the client's life style?

   c. Do the strategies help the client change behaviors in an efficient manner?

   d. Did I use appropriate verbal and nonverbal interviewing skills?

   e. Did I use appropriate counseling skills?

   f. What changes would I make?

Answers to Review of Chapter 6

1. a. Social pressures.

   b. Giving up old eating habits.

   c. Avoiding unpalatable commercial substitutes.

2. a. Complex carbohydrates.

   b. Simple carbohydrates.

3. a. Tailoring the eating pattern.

   b. Staging the diet instruction.

   c. Changing behaviors for social occasions.

   d. Involving the family.

4. a. Ask questions to elicit thought patterns surrounding the problem.

   b. Encourage food substitutes and positive thinking.

   c. The rationale is consistent with information presented by the client.

5. a. Were changes in eating pattern approached gradually and was the gradual approach successful?

   b. Was positive thinking used to try to eliminate eating problems on social occasions and how well did it work?

6. a. Was the assessment adequate in identifying potential eating problems?

   b. Was the new diet pattern tailored to client needs?

   c. Was the use of nonverbal and verbal interviewing skill appropriate?

Answers to Review of Chapter 7

1. a. Too many changes at one time.

   b. Social pressures.

   c. Giving up old eating habits.

   d. Unpalatable commercial substitutes.

2. a. Protein.
    b. Potassium.
    c. Sodium.
    d. Fluid.
3. a. Tailoring.
    b. Staging.
    c. Behavior change for social occasions.
    d. Family involvement.
4. There are many correct answers to this question. One basic strategy is to initiate added spouse involvement in the interview. If the wife is given a sense of belonging to the dietary change process, she may become a more positive influence on her husband.
5. a. Did the dietary changes fit in with the client's life style?
    b. Was the problem solved gradually?
    c. Was coping with social situations easier?
    d. Did family involvement increase?
    e. Is the family providing positive reinforcement?
6. a. Did the assessment point out problem areas?
    b. Was the eating pattern designed to allow for the client's current life style?
    c. Were the strategies efficient?
    d. Were verbal and nonverbal interviewing skills appropriate?
    e. Were counseling skills appropriate?

Answers to Review of Chapter 8

1. a. Loss of familiar flavors.
    b. Limited food choices.
    c. Changing old habits.
    d. Unpalatable commercial substitutes.
2. a. Collect data on the sodium content of the baseline diet.
    b. Identify the general problem.
    c. Identify inappropriate eating patterns and possible solutions.
3. a. Tailoring.
    b. Staging.
    c. Flavoring substitutes.
    d. Altering eating style through family involvement.

4. One of many areas to assess is family involvement. If the family members' attitudes are negative toward the sodium restriction, an increase in their involvement is a possible first step. By reviewing baseline information it may be possible to substitute foods low in sodium for cheese and cold cuts. The client and counselor can build a self-reward system when low-sodium foods are eaten and high-sodium foods avoided.

5. a. Was the goal of eliminating extremely high-sodium food reached?
   b. Have the reinforcers helped change the client's eating patterns?
   c. Are social occasions less of a problem?
   d. Does the family provide needed positive reinforcement?

6. a. Was assessment of baseline sodium intake adequate?
   b. Was life style taken into consideration in staging the diet?
   c. Were the strategies efficient?
   d. Were appropriate counseling skills used?

Answers to Review of Chapter 9

1. a. Food preferences.
   b. Number of meals per day.

2. a. Tailoring.
   b. Staging.
   c. Family involvement.

3. Many strategies are possible. One is to stimulate more family involvement. If the family could help Mrs. J. by doing some of her pressure-producing jobs, she might be able to work small frequent meals into her life style.

4. a. Does the bland eating pattern fit into the client's life style?
   b. Was the dietary change efficient and successful?
   c. Does the family provide needed positive reinforcement?

5. a. Was the assessment adequate to help in staging the diet?
   b. Did staging take into account the client's previous life style?
   c. Were appropriate verbal and nonverbal interviewing skills used?

Answers to Review of Chapter 10

1. a. Reinforce and practice in the new environment.
   b. Promote stimulus generalization.
   c. Build in resistance to extinction.
   d. Practice new behaviors sufficiently.
   e. Promote social support.

2. a. Are there things going on in your life that may cause this?
    b. If "yes," what are they?
    c. Has the intervening event passed?
3. Check with the client to determine the most useful strategy used in the past to maintain adherence. Reinstitute that plan and monitor behavior.

Index

A

ABC behavioral model, 68
Acid-neutralizing effect, 210
Action-seeking behavior, 46
Adherence, diet, 45, 74-76, 80, 96, 145, 146, 159, 161, 173, 174, 175, 176, 177, 178, 189, 190, 199, 211, 221, 223, 225
  client's role, 75
  clinic's role, 75
  counselor's role, 75
  deterrents to, 12
  inducements for, 12-13
  objective and subjective data, 77
  predictors, 76-77
  regimen's role, 76
  tools, 121, 122, 147, 148, 163, 164, 179, 180, 200, 201, 213, 214
Affective focus, 40
Affective messages, 44
Affective state, 68
Algorithm, 223
Alternate response, 94
Aluminum hydroxide, 173
Anorexigenic agents, 118
Antecedent, 29, 68, 158, 191, 194, 222
Anxiety, client, 78
Assertive thoughts, 86, 87
Assessment factors, 111

Assessment phase of counseling, 13-14, 16-17, 110-113, 137-138, 156, 174, 187-190, 209-210
Attributing response, 46-47
Attributing statement, 50
  See also Attributing response
Authier, J., 51, 52
Authoritarian role, 7, 26, 27

B

Baseline data, 73, 189, 211
Baseline information, 93
  See also Baseline data
Behavior change steps, 77-78
Behavioral being, 10
Behavioral chart, 73, 92, 247
Behavioral goal, 69
Behavioral log, 73, 92, 247, 249, 251
Biochemical analysis, 96
Blood urea nitrogen (BUN), 177
Brammer, L.M., 27, 43, 50
Body fat, 111
Body image, 10, 18
Body weight, 111

C

Calipers, 111
Calorie counting, 113

267

D

About the Author

LINDA G. SNETSELAAR graduated from Iowa State University with a Bachelor of Science Degree in Food and Nutrition in 1972. She did a dietetic internship at the University of Iowa and became a registered dietitian in 1973. Dr. Snetselaar received a Master of Science Degree from the University of Iowa in Nutrition in 1975, and a Doctor of Philosophy Degree in Instructional Design (Health Sciences Education) in 1983.

She has worked as a clinical dietitian instructing patients on modified diets, and as a research nutritionist counseling cardiovascular patients on diet and medication. As head research nutritionist she directed the Foods and Nutrition Resource Center for the Lipid Research Clinic's Coronary Primary Prevention Trial (a clinical trial funded by the National Institutes of Health). Presently she is involved in a nationally funded study, the Diabetes Complication and Control Trial.

She has directed seven NIH- (National Institutes of Health) funded workshops on counseling skills applied to nutrition. She has also given numerous talks on the topic. In 1978 Dr. Snetselaar was named Recognized Young Dietitian of the Year in Iowa and received the honor of being named an Outstanding Young Woman in America for 1982.